# Ladders to Success on the Illinois Standards

## SCIENCE, LEVEL C

Triumph Learning®

Ladders to Success on the Illinois Standards, Science, Level C
130IL
ISBN-10: 1-60471-061-6
ISBN-13: 978-1-60471-061-8

Content Consultant: Carl Proujan
Content Development: Mazer Creative Services
Cover Image: © Mark Collins/Deborah Wolfe Ltd.

**Triumph Learning**® 136 Madison Avenue, 7th Floor, New York, NY 10016
Kevin McAliley, President and Chief Executive Officer

Printed in the United States of America.

10 9 8 7 6 5 4 3 2 1

# Ladders to Success on the Illinois Standards

## SCIENCE, LEVEL C

# TABLE OF CONTENTS

## Performance Descriptors

**Stage B:** 11A-1 to 11A-4; 11B-1 to 11B-5; 13A-1, 13A-2
**Stage C:** 11A-1 to 11A-4; 13A-1, 13A-2
**Stage D:** 11A-1 to 11A-3; 13A-1, 13A-2

**Stage B:** 11A-5, 11A-6
**Stage C:** 11A-5
**Stage D:** 11A-4, 11A-5, 11B-4, 11B-6

**Stage B:** 12D-1, 12D-2
**Stage C:** 12C-1, 12D-1, 12D-2
**Stage D:** 12D-1, 12D-2

**Stage B:** 12C-2; **Stage C:** 12C-2
**Stage D:** 12C-2

**Stage B:** 12C-1; **Stage C:** 12C-1
**Stage D:** 12C-1

**Stage C:** 12A-1, 12B-1, 12B-2
**Stage D:** 12B-2

**Stage B:** 12A-1, 12B-1, 12B-2
**Stage C:** 12B-1, 12B-2
**Stage D:** 12A-1 to 12A-4; 12B-1

**Stage B:** 12F-1, 12F-2
**Stage C:** 12E-1, 12F-1, 12F-2
**Stage D:** 12E-1, 12F-1, 12F-2

**Stage C:** 12E-2; **Stage D:** 12E-2

**Stage B:** 12E-2; **Stage D:** 12E-1

# CHECK YOUR UNDERSTANDING

Read each question carefully. Decide which choice is the best answer. Choose the best answer for each question. Mark your answer on your answer sheet. If you do not know the answer to a question, you can skip it and come back to it later.

1. What do you do when you observe something?

   A. You write a description of it.

   B. You use your senses to learn about it.

   C. You guess why something has occurred.

   D. You find the answer to a question.

2. All living things

   A. know how to swim.

   B. reproduce.

   C. make their own food.

   D. grow from seeds.

3. Which living thing is a producer?

   A. a fish

   B. a dog

   C. a turtle

   D. a tree

4. Which living thing is a decomposer?

   A. a mushroom

   B. an octopus

   C. an ant

   D. a rose bush

5. When you use a simple machine, you

   A. increase the amount of force.

   B. need to do less work.

   C. need to do more work.

   D. make work easier.

6. You are using a wheel and axle when you

   A. throw a basketball.

   B. twist a doorknob.

   C. open a box.

   D. use a keyboard.

7. A variable is

   A. a change in how an experiment is done.

   B. something that can change a test result.

   C. a result that supports the hypothesis.

   D. a change in the data and the hypothesis.

8. Which of these organisms is extinct?

   A. humans

   B. dinosaurs

   C. seagulls

   D. dolphins

9. Stored energy is also called

   A. motion.

   B. heat energy.

   C. kinetic energy.

   D. potential energy.

10. How long does it take Earth to revolve once around the sun?

    A. about one month

    B. about one day

    C. about one week

    D. about one year

11. Wind speed is measured with a(n)

   A.  anemometer.

   B.  barometer.

   C.  wind vane.

   D.  thermometer.

12. A large sheet of moving ice is called

   A.  erosion.

   B.  an earthquake.

   C.  a glacier.

   D.  precipitation.

13. What is an experiment?

   A.  a scientific guess

   B.  something you can measure

   C.  a controlled test

   D.  an observation

14. When you keep track of what you observe, you are

   A.  observing.

   B.  asking a question.

   C.  recording.

   D.  concluding.

15. Plants make their own food. Plants are

   A.  producers.

   B.  consumers.

   C.  decomposers.

   D.  predators.

16. If it is winter in the Northern Hemisphere, what season is it in the Southern Hemisphere?

   A. summer

   B. winter

   C. spring

   D. fall

17. Which describes evaporation?

   A. Liquid water changes to water vapor.

   B. Ice changes to water vapor.

   C. Ice changes to liquid water.

   D. Water vapor changes to liquid water.

18. A long crack in Earth's crust is called a(n)

   A. volcano.

   B. earthquake.

   C. crater.

   D. fault.

19. When you plan an experiment, a control is

   A. a data table.

   B. a testable hypothesis.

   C. something you allow to change.

   D. something you keep from changing.

20. Measurements are

   A. a kind of experiment.

   B. a kind of observation.

   C. a way of checking your data.

   D. a way of displaying your data.

21. If you are observing a regular change in something, you are probably observing a

    **A.**    line graph.

    **B.**    conclusion.

    **C.**    pattern.

    **D.**    data table.

22. Which tool would you use to find out how long it takes to climb a stairway?

    **A.**    a balance

    **B.**    a meterstick

    **C.**    a watch

    **D.**    a thermometer

23. Hugo measured and compared the masses of two toy trucks. What property was he investigating?

    **A.**    the amount of matter in the trucks

    **B.**    the materials that make up trucks

    **C.**    how hot or cold trucks are

    **D.**    the amount of space trucks take up

24. A canyon is usually formed by

    **A.**    a river

    **B.**    a landslide

    **C.**    an earthquake

    **D.**    a volcano

**Use the picture below to answer question 25.**

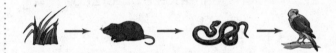

25. The picture shows a desert food chain. What is the role of the grass in this food chain?

    **A.**    The grass provides a habitat for the hawk.

    **B.**    The grass provides energy for the snake.

    **C.**    The grass provides energy for the hawk.

    **D.**    The grass provides energy for the mouse.

26. How long does it take for the moon to revolve once around Earth?

    A. about one month

    B. about one day

    C. about one week

    D. about one year

27. Motion is

    A. a change of position.

    B. a change of speed.

    C. only an up and down movement.

    D. only a back and forth movement.

28. What is a conclusion?

    A. an observation

    B. an answer to a question

    C. a way of interpreting data

    D. a line graph made from data

29. Fossils are

    A. preserved remains or evidence of once-living things.

    B. living things

    C. rocks.

    D. tree sap.

30. Which adaptation helps a fish move through water?

    A. gills

    B. eyes

    C. fins

    D. bright colors

31. An opening in Earth's surface from which melted rock flows is called

    A. a fault.

    B. an earthquake.

    C. a volcano.

    D. a landslide.

32. What is weather?

    A. the amount of rain that falls during a day

    B. what the air is like around you

    C. the amount of water vapor in the clouds

    D. the speed of wind

33. Why might you want to investigate something?

    A. to find the answer to a question

    B. to gather data that you can put in a table

    C. to see how many variables there are

    D. to decide which parts of an experiment to control

34. When you use force to move an object a distance,

    A. work is being done.

    B. something changes direction.

    C. there is no opposing force.

    D. you are using a machine.

35. Look at this bird's foot.

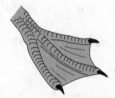

Where does this bird spend most of its time?

    A. in a river or lake

    B. in a desert

    C. in a field

    D. in a dry canyon

36. A process that makes rocks wear down or break apart is called

   A.   erosion.

   B.   acid rain.

   C.   weathering.

   D.   dissolving.

37. Which of the following would you use to measure the volume of a liquid?

   A.   a meterstick

   B.   a balance

   C.   a measuring cup

   D.   a spring scale

38. Shana placed a cup of water in a warm place. One week later, no water was left in the cup. What probably happened?

   A.   The liquid water changed to a gas.

   B.   The liquid water changed to a solid.

   C.   The water leaked out of the cup.

   D.   The water spilled from the cup.

39. Which is another name for energy of motion?

   A.   heat energy

   B.   electrical energy

   C.   kinetic energy

   D.   potential energy

40. When you burn firewood, you are converting

   A.   chemical energy into heat energy.

   B.   kinetic energy into heat energy.

   C.   sound energy into light energy.

   D.   mechanical energy into potential energy.

41. Water is constantly moving from Earth's surface into the air and back again. This never-ending process is called the

    A. weather cycle.

    B. condensation.

    C. water cycle.

    D. precipitation.

42. What is volume?

    A. the amount of matter in an object

    B. the materials that make up matter

    C. how hot or cold matter is

    D. the amount of space an object takes up

43. A push or a pull is also called a

    A. motion.

    B. force.

    C. speed.

    D. position.

44. You go to the beach on a sunny day. The sand is hot on your feet. Where did this heat come from?

    A. electricity

    B. water

    C. fossil fuels

    D. the sun

45. Falling rain or snow is called

    A. evaporation.

    B. condensation.

    C. sublimation.

    D. precipitation.

46. Which will cause liquid water to change to a solid?

    A. warming

    B. heating

    C. freezing

    D. dripping

47. How many poles does Earth have?

    A. one

    B. two

    C. three

    D. four

48. Which of these is MOST likely to become a fossil?

    A. a dinosaur's skin

    B. a worm

    C. a fish bone

    D. an insect's wing

49. Which statement about energy is true?

    A. Energy never changes.

    B. Energy can be a solid, liquid, or gas.

    C. Energy exists only as heat or electrical energy.

    D. Energy can change from one form to another.

50. How long does it take Earth to spin once on its axis?

    A. one month

    B. one day

    C. one week

    D. one year

# Investigating

## LESSON 1: **THE BASICS**

### KEY CONCEPTS

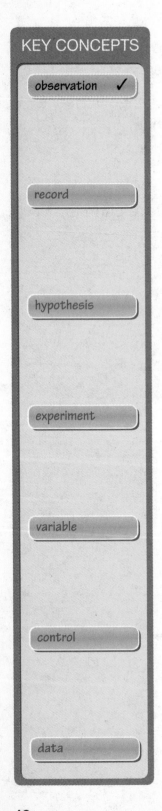

observation ✓

record

hypothesis

experiment

variable

control

data

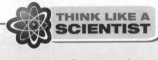
**THINK LIKE A SCIENTIST**

You live on a farm with your family. Every summer the corn grows tall and green. You remember hearing people say that corn should be "knee high by the Fourth of July." But it is late July now. The plants just reach your knees. At this time last year, they were much taller.

You know that plants need sunlight and water to grow. You know that the same amount of sunlight fell on the fields this year as last year. You also find that the amount of rain was the same both years.

You wonder: What caused the corn to be shorter this year? What is different about this year?

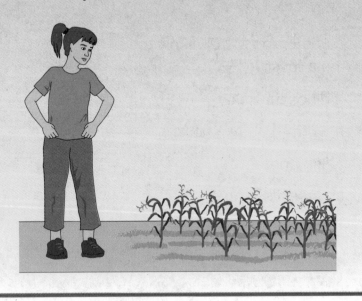

## Observing and Asking Questions

Science is about investigating. Most investigations start with an observation. An **observation** is something you see, hear, smell, taste, or touch. A puzzling observation makes you ask a question. When you investigate, you look for answers to the question.

For example, you observed that the corn on your farm is shorter than usual this year. You also observed that the amount of sun and rain have not changed from last year to this year.

How did you make your observations? You used your senses. And you may have used tools. What kind of tool can you use to measure rainfall? You could have used a rain gauge.

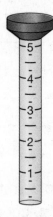

You then recorded the measurements. Keeping records allows you to compare measurements. That's how you can compare rainfall in different years.

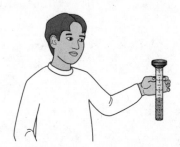

When you use a rain gauge, you look at the markings to see how much rain has fallen. Then you record that measurement.

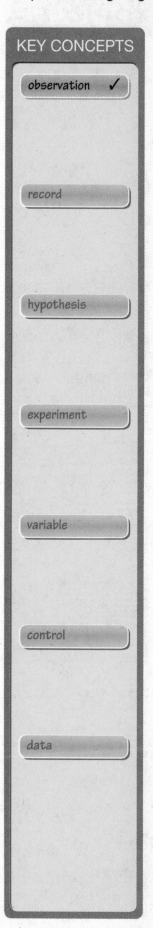

KEY CONCEPTS

observation ✓

record

hypothesis

experiment

variable

control

data

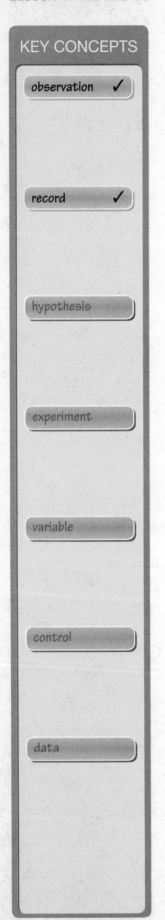

KEY CONCEPTS

observation ✓

record ✓

hypothesis

experiment

variable

control

data

When you **record** an observation, you keep track of what you observe. You can write a description. You can draw pictures. You can also write measurements in a table.

**Last Year's Rainfall**

| Month | Precipitation in Inches |
|---|---|
| April | 4 |
| May | 5 |
| June | 4 |
| July | 3 |
| August | 2 |
| September | 3 |

You are sure the same amount of rain fell this year as the year before. How are you so sure? You check the rainfall records that scientists keep. You find those records in an almanac or on the Internet.

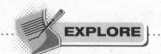

Look at the pictures of the three rain gauges. Write how much rain each one has collected.

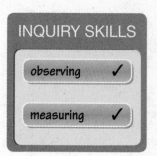
| Rain gauge | Measurements |
|:---:|:---:|
| 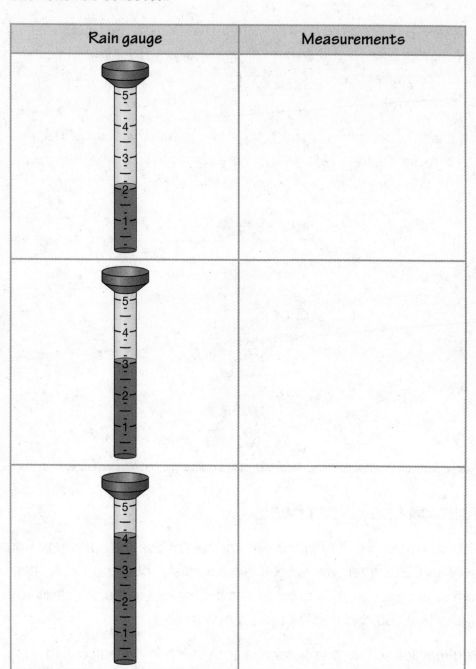 | |
| | |
| | |

# LESSON 2: **BUILDING ON THE BASICS**

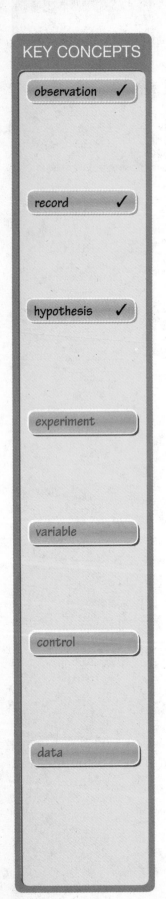

## KEY CONCEPTS

observation ✓

record ✓

hypothesis ✓

experiment

variable

control

data

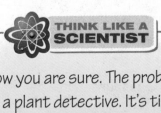

**THINK LIKE A SCIENTIST**

Now you are sure. The problem is not lack of rain or sun. It is time to be a plant detective. It's time to solve the corn mystery! To figure out the problem, you need to find out what else can affect how a plant grows.

Besides water and sunlight, a plant needs soil. You are puzzled. This is the same soil in which healthy corn plants have always grown. It looks the same, but could the soil be the problem?

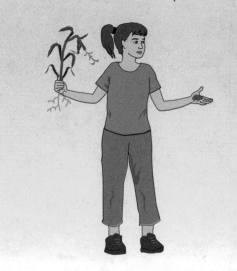

## Testing the Hypothesis

You can make a scientific guess. You can guess the answer to your question. But when you work like a scientist, you need to be able to test your guess. You need to see if it makes sense. A scientific guess that you can test is called a **hypothesis**.

You may know that plants take in something in the soil called nutrients. All living things need nutrients to live and grow. You get nutrients from the food you eat.

Let's say this is your hypothesis: The corn plants are short because the soil doesn't hold enough nutrients. Now you need to test your hypothesis. One way to test a hypothesis is to perform an experiment.

An **experiment** is a controlled test. What does that mean?

Say you want to know whether a wooden or metal bat makes a ball travel farther. To find out, you hit a ball with a metal bat. Then you hit a ball with a wooden bat.

Suppose the ball you hit with the metal bat travels farther. Does this mean metal bats hit balls farther than wooden bats? Maybe, but maybe not. Other things might make a ball travel farther.

The only way you can find out whether the material the bats are made of affects the distance the ball travels is to perform an experiment.

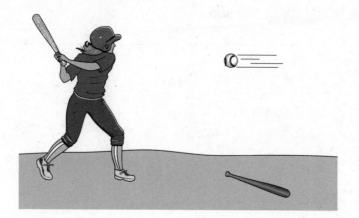

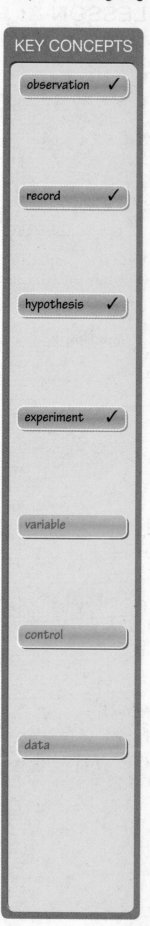

KEY CONCEPTS

observation ✓

record ✓

hypothesis ✓

experiment ✓

variable

control

data

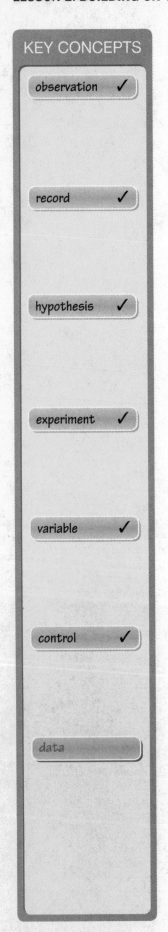

KEY CONCEPTS

observation ✓

record ✓

hypothesis ✓

experiment ✓

variable ✓

control ✓

data

# Variables

In a controlled experiment, you have to keep all but one variable the same. A **variable** is something that can change a result, such as how far a ball will travel.

The kind of bat is a variable. The speed of your swing is a variable. The type of ball is also a variable. Each of these variables might affect how far the ball travels. You want to know the effect of the kind of bat. That means you have to control all the variables EXCEPT the kind of bat.

You **control** a variable by keeping it from changing. Using each bat, you must swing with the same speed. And you must use the same ball with each bat. Then you can be fairly sure that the distance the ball travels is changed only by the type of bat you used.

What about your corn experiment? You need to control everything except the nutrients in the soil.

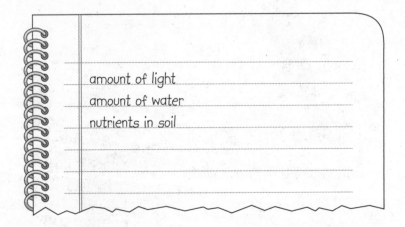

amount of light
amount of water
nutrients in soil

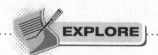

Below are two hypotheses. In the space provided, describe an experiment that would test each hypothesis. Then list the variables and tell which ones you have to control.

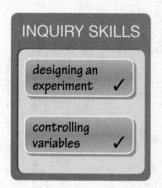

INQUIRY SKILLS

designing an experiment ✓

controlling variables ✓

**Hypothesis**     *If a plant gets more sunlight, it will grow faster.*
**Experiment**

_____

_____

_____

**Variables**

_____

_____

**Variables to control**

_____

_____

**Hypothesis**     *If a plant gets too little water, it will grow slower.*
**Experiment**

_____

_____

_____

**Variables**

_____

_____

**Variables to control**

_____

_____

## KEY CONCEPTS

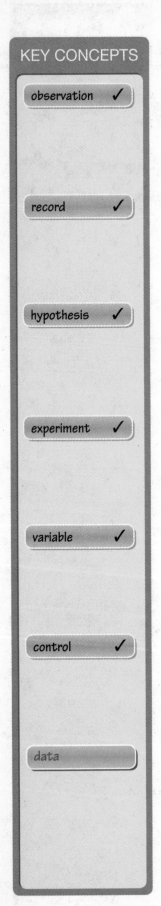

- observation ✓
- record ✓
- hypothesis ✓
- experiment ✓
- variable ✓
- control ✓
- data

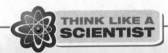

**THINK LIKE A SCIENTIST**

You wonder what kind of experiment would best test your hypothesis. You think about the variables. The amount of sunlight and rain are variables that you need to control. But there is no light switch on the sun and no faucet for the rain. How will you measure and control the variables of light and water?

The cornfield is too big to put into a lab. You need something smaller, a model. How can you make a model of the cornfield and control the variables, all at the same time?

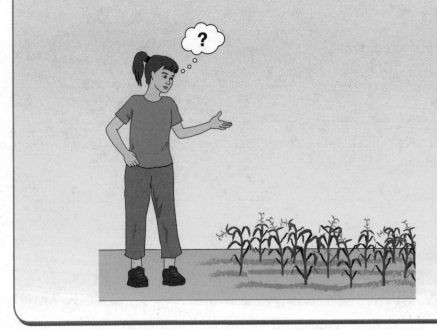

# Testing and Interpreting Data

Sometimes when you experiment you need to use a model instead of the real thing.

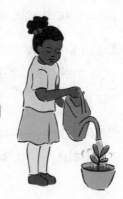

Say you wanted to find out how water pollution affects plants growing on the banks of a river. You would not pollute the river to find out. You could add pollutants to a cup of water. Then you could pour the water on a potted plant. The polluted water and potted plant are models for the real things.

**Start of Experiment**          **One Week Later**

Pot 1          Pot 2                    Pot 1          Pot 2

You model the cornfield by planting corn sprouts in two pots. The sprouts are the same size. So are the pots.

You put the same amount of soil from the cornfield in each pot. You put the pots next to each other on a window sill. That way, they will get the same amount of sunlight. You also give each plant the same amount of water each day.

Everything is the same, except one thing. You add some fertilizer to the second pot. Fertilizer contains nutrients that help plants grow.

All the variables are controlled, or the same, EXCEPT for the fertilizer.

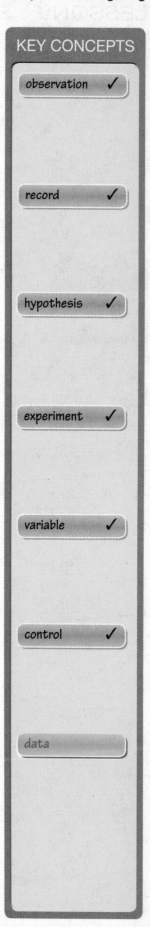

KEY CONCEPTS

observation ✓

record ✓

hypothesis ✓

experiment ✓

variable ✓

control ✓

data

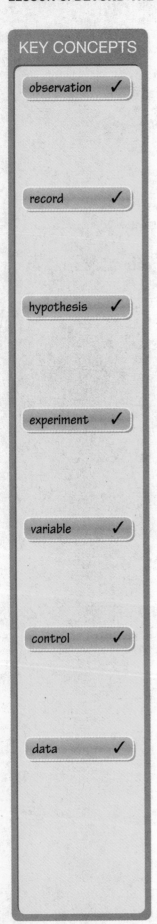

Starting on the third day of your investigation, you measure each plant every day. You record the measurements in your journal. The measurements are called data.

**Data** are observations. In your experiment, the measurements you make are data. Organizing the data makes them easier to understand.

You can organize the data in a table. Then you can make a graph of the data. A graph is a kind of picture of the data.

|  | Plant 1 | Plant 2 |
|---|---|---|
|  | No fertilizer | With fertilizer |
|  | Plant height in millimeters... |  |
| ...on Day 3 | 25 | 25 |
| ...on Day 4 | 31 | 45 |
| ...on Day 5 | 44 | 64 |
| ...on Day 6 | 63 | 82 |
| ...on Day 7 | 76 | 102 |

Look at the graph. It shows you that the soil in the cornfield lacked enough nutrients to make the plants grow tall. The graph tells you that your hypothesis was a good scientific guess.

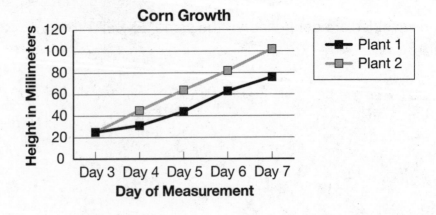

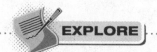 **EXPLORE**

The data you gather in an experiment will not mean much unless you can interpret them. The chart below shows the results of two investigations. Make a graph of the data in the space provided. Then explain what your graph means.

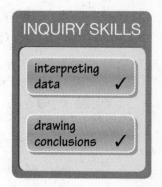

INQUIRY SKILLS

interpreting data ✓

drawing conclusions ✓

Best soil temperature for corn seeds to sprout

50° F ......... 22 days to sprout
59° F ......... 12 days
68° F ........... 7 days
77° F ........... 4 days
86° F ........... 4 days

**Best Soil Temperature to Sprout Corn**

Number of Days for Corn Seed to Sprout

30
25
20
15
10
5
0

10 20 30 40 50 60 70 80 90 100

Soil Temperature in Degrees Fahrenheit

What does the graph tell you about how temperature affects sprouting time?

Price of a bag of popcorn
January 2008 ..... $ .89
February 2008 .... $ .96
March 2008 ......... $ .98
April 2008 ............. $ .98
May 2008 .............. $ 1.09
June 2008 ............. $ 1.01

**Price of Bag of Popcorn**

$1.10
$1.05
$1.00
$0.95
$0.90
$0.85
$0.80

Jan  Feb  Mar  Apr  May  Jun

What does the graph tell you about how the price of popcorn changes during the year?

# PUTTING IT ALL TOGETHER

**You are now ready to show you understand the key concepts covered in this topic. Read each question. Circle the letter of the best answer.**

1. Which is an example of observing?

   A. riding a bicycle

   B. eating dinner

   C. watching someone cook

   D. knitting a sweater

2. Which is a type of observing?

   A. measuring temperature

   B. drawing a picture

   C. recording information

   D. making a table or a graph

3. What is a hypothesis?

   A. an observation

   B. an investigation

   C. a test

   D. a scientific guess

4. Which is an example of recording?

   A. watching a butterfly

   B. drawing a butterfly

   C. singing about a butterfly

   D. reading about a butterfly

5. How do you test a hypothesis?

   A. gather data

   B. make a graph

   C. perform an experiment

   D. record results

6. What is a variable?

   A. something that can change a result

   B. an experiment that changes

   C. a type of observation

   D. a way of making measurements

7. What is the purpose of an investigation?

   A. to keep records

   B. to gather data

   C. to answer a question or test a hypothesis

   D. to form a hypothesis

**Use the table to answer questions 8 and 9.**

Sarah counted living things in a meadow during four summers. She made this table from her data.

| SUMMERS IN A MEADOW | | | | |
|---|---|---|---|---|
| | 2005 | 2006 | 2007 | 2008 |
| crickets | 400 | 350 | 327 | 298 |
| birds | 60 | 75 | 77 | 82 |
| mice | 260 | 253 | 260 | 280 |
| snakes | 9 | 9 | 8 | 7 |

8. Which is true?

   A. From 2005 to 2008, the number of mice steadily went up.

   B. From 2005 to 2008, the number of crickets went down each year.

   C. From 2005 to 2008, the number of snakes went up each year.

   D. More birds were counted in 2005 than in 2008.

9. Which statement is true?

   A. As the number of birds went up, the number of crickets also went up.

   B. As the number of crickets went down, the number of birds also went down.

   C. As the number of birds went up, the number of crickets went down.

   D. There is no connection between the numbers of birds and crickets.

10. Elliot wants to know if the temperature in his classroom changes during the day. He plans to measure the temperature once every hour. What should Elliot do as he takes each measurement?

    A. Try to keep the temperature data in his head.

    B. Record the time and temperature in a chart.

    C. Remember the time that each measurement was taken.

    D. Compare the new measurement only to the last measurement.

# Working with Data

## LESSON 1: **THE BASICS**

**KEY CONCEPTS**

experiment ✓

data

table

graph

interpret data

pattern

conclusion

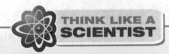
**THINK LIKE A SCIENTIST**

You are about to run in a footrace. You will run all the way around a soccer field. Ready! Set! Go! You are off and running! You run as fast as you can. You reach the halfway point. You feel your heart beating fast. You run even faster! At last you cross the finish line. Your heart is really pounding! You catch your breath and your heartbeat begins to slow.

You can tell that running makes your heart beat quickly. But does your heart keep beating faster and faster the farther you run?

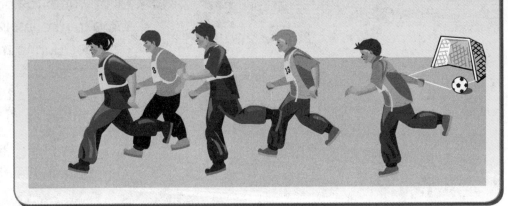

## Planning The Experiment

Your heart rate is the number of times your heart beats in a minute. You know that running raises your heart rate. But you want to find out whether your heart rate keeps rising as you run. To find out, you decide to do an experiment. An **experiment** is a controlled test.

Your friends Jeff and Kisha will help you. You decide to run today's race again. You will run more slowly. But you will run five times as far!

Jeff will measure your heart rate each time you complete a lap. He will put his fingers on your wrist. Then he can feel your heartbeat through your blood vessels. This is called your pulse. He will count the number of beats in ten seconds. Then he will multiply the number by six. This will tell him the number of beats in one minute.

Scientists use tools in experiments to help them observe and measure. What kind of tool would help Jeff measure your pulse?

A watch would be a useful tool. Jeff can use the watch to measure ten seconds of time.

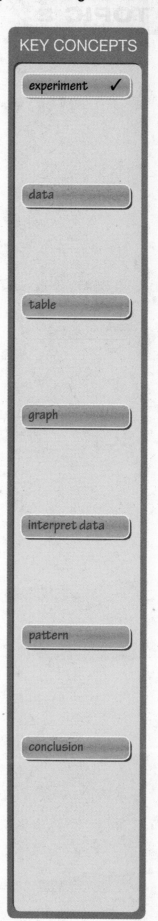

KEY CONCEPTS

experiment ✓

data

table

graph

interpret data

pattern

conclusion

31

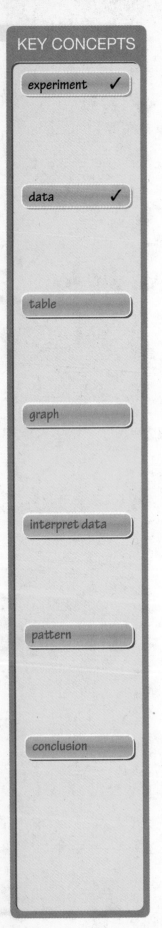

KEY CONCEPTS

experiment ✓

data ✓

table

graph

interpret data

pattern

conclusion

By taking measurements, Jeff is gathering data. **Data** are observations. Measurements are one kind of observation. So measurements of your heart rate are data. Kisha will record the data from the experiment. You can use those data to answer your question about how running affects your heart rate.

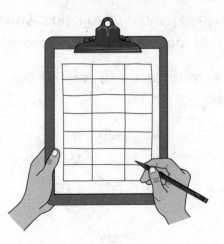

You plan to run five laps around the soccer field. Does this mean that Kisha will write down five measurements? No, she will write down six measurements. First she will record your heart rate before you start to run. Then she will record a measurement every time you finish a lap.

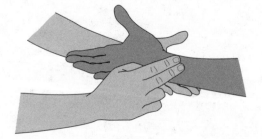

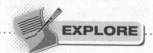 **EXPLORE**

Work with a partner to gather data about exercise and heart rate. Take your partner's pulse twice by using the steps below. First, take your partner's pulse after your partner has been resting. Then, take your partner's pulse just after your partner exercises for two minutes. Exercising might be running in place.

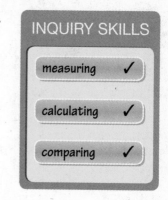

**INQUIRY SKILLS**

| measuring | ✓ |
| calculating | ✓ |
| comparing | ✓ |

1. Put two fingers over your partner's wrist as shown in the drawing on page 32. Move your fingers until you can feel a pulse.

2. Count the number of beats for 10 seconds. Use the second hand of a watch or clock to measure seconds.

3. Write the number of beats in the first column of the table.

4. Multiply the number by 6. Write the product in the last column. This is your partner's heart rate.

5. Take your partner's pulse again right after your partner exercises.

| | Number of Beats in Ten Seconds | Multiply by Six | Heart Rate (Beats per Minute) |
|---|---|---|---|
| While resting | | × 6 = | |
| After exercise | | × 6 = | |

Compare the heart rates. What difference do you find?

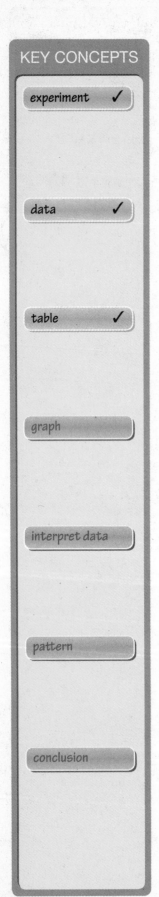

KEY CONCEPTS

experiment ✓

data ✓

table ✓

graph

interpret data

pattern

conclusion

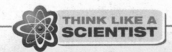

**THINK LIKE A SCIENTIST**

Now you are ready to do the experiment. You lace up your running shoes. Jeff takes your pulse before you begin. And Kisha writes down your heart rate. Then off you go! After each lap, you stop for a moment to let Jeff measure your heart rate. Then, before you can catch your breath, you start running again.

You are very tired, but you have run all five laps. Your heart is pounding. Jeff takes your pulse for the sixth time.

The experiment has gone well. Kisha has plenty of data. How has she chosen to record the data? How will she organize them so you can easily see what they tell?

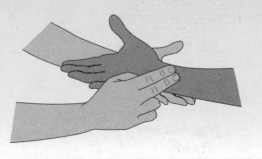

## Working with Data

Kisha has made a table to hold the data from the experiment. A **table** is a chart for listing numbers and facts. A table has columns and rows. Each column and row is labeled. The labels tell what data should go in that column or row.

Using a table is a good way to record the data from your experiment.

Here is Kisha's table with the experiment's data.

| PULSE AFTER EACH LAP | | |
|---|---|---|
| Number of Laps | Heart Beats in Ten Seconds | Heart Rate |
| 0 | 14 | 84 |
| 1 | 20 | 120 |
| 2 | 22 | 132 |
| 3 | 23 | 138 |
| 4 | 23 | 138 |
| 5 | 23 | 138 |

Another way to show data is to put them in a graph. A **graph** is a kind of picture that can show how one action can cause a change in another action.

Kisha decided to put the data in a graph. Her graph will show how the action of your running caused a change in your heart rate.

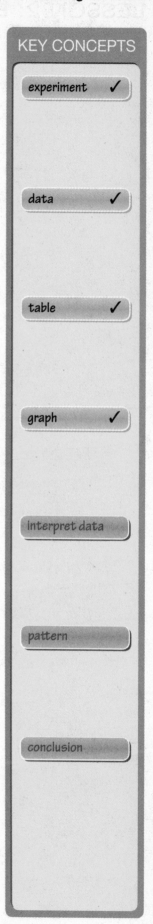

KEY CONCEPTS

experiment ✓

data ✓

table ✓

graph ✓

interpret data

pattern

conclusion

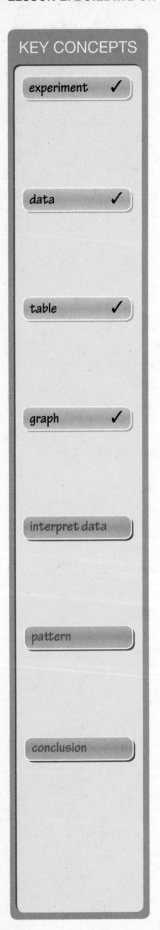

KEY CONCEPTS

experiment ✓

data ✓

table ✓

graph ✓

interpret data

pattern

conclusion

Here is Kisha's graph showing the data.

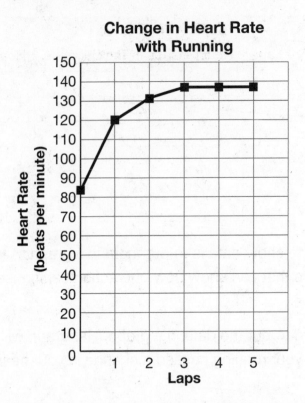

The numbers along the bottom stand for the laps that you ran. The numbers going up the side stand for your heart rate.

This kind of graph is called a line graph. It shows the data as dots, or points. The points tell how fast your heart was beating after each lap. A line connects the points.

What was your heart rate at the end of one lap? Find the number 1 along the bottom of the graph. Then find the dot above it. Look at the number directly to the left of the dot. You can see that your heart rate was 120 beats per minute. That's how fast your heart was beating at the end of the first lap.

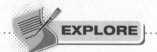 **EXPLORE**

The table shows the usual number of times that the heart beats each minute in young people of different ages. The data are for people who are resting.

Below the table is a grid that you will use to make a graph of the data in the table. You will make the graph by using data from the table. Two data points are missing from the grid. Find the data for those missing points in the table. Add those two points to the grid. Then connect the lines to make your graph.

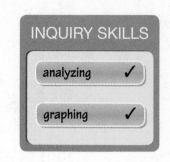

| Age (years) | Usual Heart Rate (beats per minute) |
|:---:|:---:|
| 1–3 | 130 |
| 4–5 | 100 |
| 6–8 | 100 |
| 9–11 | 88 |
| 12–16 | 80 |
| >16 | 70 |

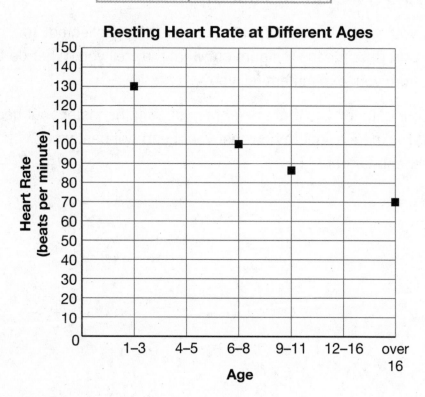

# LESSON 3: **BEYOND THE BASICS**

## KEY CONCEPTS

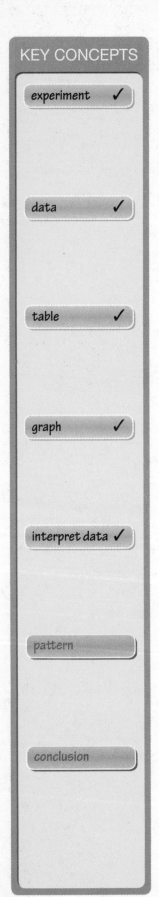

experiment ✓

data ✓

table ✓

graph ✓

interpret data ✓

pattern

conclusion

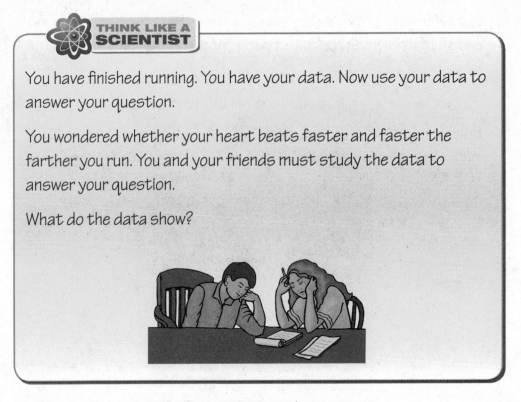

**THINK LIKE A SCIENTIST**

You have finished running. You have your data. Now use your data to answer your question.

You wondered whether your heart beats faster and faster the farther you run. You and your friends must study the data to answer your question.

What do the data show?

## Making Conclusions about Data

Now you must interpret the data your team has collected. To **interpret data** means to figure out what they tell you. What do the data from your experiment tell you?

Do your data tell you that the farther you run, the faster your heart beats? Is there a limit to how fast your heart will beat when you run farther and farther?

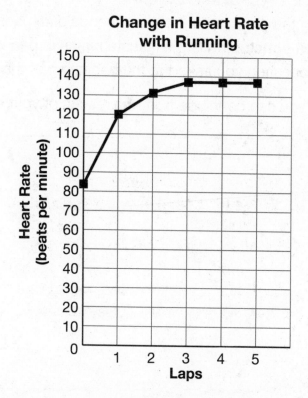

**Change in Heart Rate with Running**

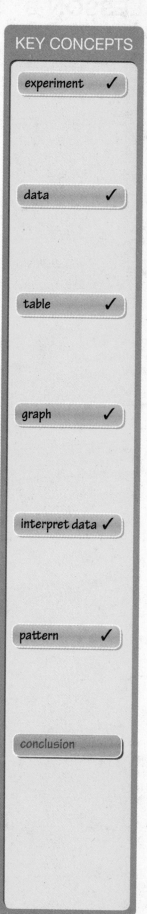

KEY CONCEPTS

experiment ✓

data ✓

table ✓

graph ✓

interpret data ✓

pattern ✓

conclusion

You and your friends study the graph. The graph is the line on the grid. You look for a pattern in the shape of the line. A **pattern** is a regular change in the line. You find a pattern in the line. It goes up very quickly between laps 0 and 2. Then it levels out.

What does this pattern mean? It means your heart rate rose rapidly from the time you started running till you finished the second lap. It also means that your heart rate stayed about the same during the rest of your run.

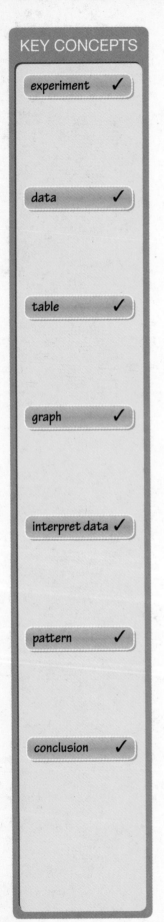

KEY CONCEPTS

experiment ✓

data ✓

table ✓

graph ✓

interpret data ✓

pattern ✓

conclusion ✓

After studying the graph, you and your friends can reach some conclusions. A **conclusion** is the last step in an experiment. It answers the question you asked at the beginning of the experiment.

Here is what you can conclude from the results of your experiment.

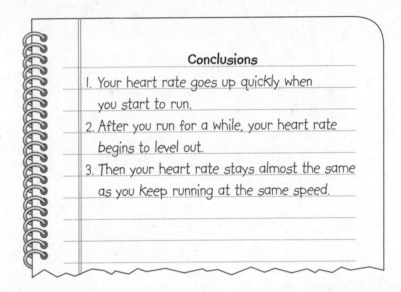

Conclusions

1. Your heart rate goes up quickly when you start to run.
2. After you run for a while, your heart rate begins to level out.
3. Then your heart rate stays almost the same as you keep running at the same speed.

Do the conclusions make sense? Your leg muscles need more oxygen when you run. Your blood carries oxygen. Your heart pumps blood to all parts of your body. That includes your legs.

So it makes sense that your heart beats faster when you run. The conclusions make sense, and they answer the question that led to your experiment.

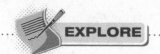 **EXPLORE**

You and your friends did another experiment. You ran at different speeds on a treadmill. Jeff took your pulse after you ran for three minutes. Kisha recorded the speed and your pulse. Then you turned up the speed and ran for another three minutes. The data are shown in the table and in the line graph. Look for patterns in the data. Then write a conclusion based on what the data show.

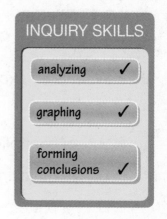

INQUIRY SKILLS

| analyzing | ✓ |
| graphing | ✓ |
| forming conclusions | ✓ |

| YOUR HEART RATE AT DIFFERENT SPEEDS | |
| --- | --- |
| Speed (miles per hour) | Heart Rate (beats per minute) |
| 0 | 75 |
| 2 | 89 |
| 4 | 111 |
| 6 | 130 |
| 8 | 148 |
| 10 | 167 |

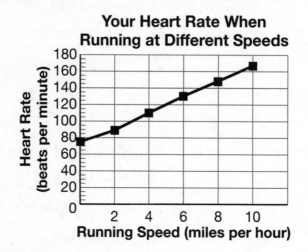

**Your Heart Rate When Running at Different Speeds**

Conclusion: _____

_____

_____

# PUTTING IT ALL TOGETHER

**You are now ready to show you understand the key concepts covered in this topic. Read each question. Circle the letter of the best answer.**

1. What is an experiment?

   A. a test

   B. a controlled test

   C. a measurement

   D. a pattern

2. You want to find out how long it takes water to boil. Which tool would you use?

   A. a scale

   B. a thermometer

   C. a ruler

   D. a watch

3. What are data?

   A. observations

   B. a set of answers

   C. an experiment

   D. conclusions

4. How are data recorded in a table?

   A. in rows and columns

   B. as a graph

   C. as a conclusion

   D. as dots connected by lines

5. What can a graph show?

   A. the plan for an experiment

   B. how one action can cause a change in another action

   C. a conclusion

   D. a table of data

6. Which name is given to a regular change in data?

   A. experiment

   B. conclusion

   C. pattern

   D. graph

**Use the graph below to answer questions 7 and 8.**

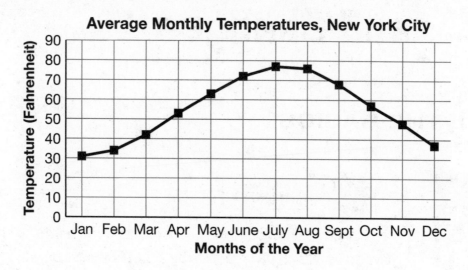

7. What is this kind of graph called?

   A. a conclusion graph

   B. a line graph

   C. a table graph

   D. a data graph

9. What are you doing when you try to figure out what data tell you?

   A. organizing data

   B. interpreting data

   C. collecting data

   D. recording data

8. What does the graph show?

   A. the number of seasons in a year

   B. what temperature is

   C. how temperature changes during a year

   D. how time changes with the season

10. What is a conclusion?

   A. an experiment

   B. a graph

   C. the last step in an experiment

   D. a record of data

# Forces, Motion, and Changes

## LESSON 1: **THE BASICS**

### KEY CONCEPTS

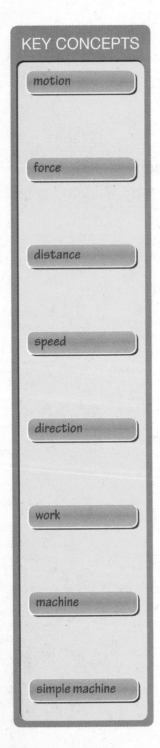

- motion
- force
- distance
- speed
- direction
- work
- machine
- simple machine

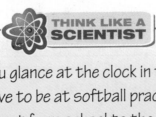 **THINK LIKE A SCIENTIST**

You glance at the clock in the school hallway. It reads 3:15! You have to be at softball practice by 3:30. You have only 15 minutes to get from school to the softball field.

"Good thing I have my rollerblades," you think. "I can use them to glide across the sidewalks. There are twelve blocks between school and the field. That means I have a lot of distance to travel in a short time. I'd better get going! But can I make it in time? What do I need to know to answer the question?"

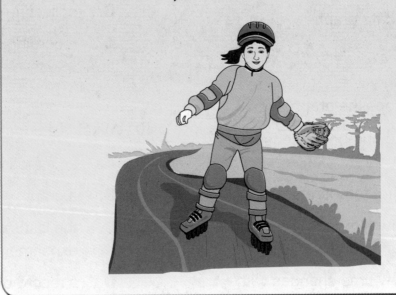

## Forces Affect Objects

To answer your question, you need to know some facts about motion. To begin with, you must know where you are and where you want to be.

You are at one position. That's your school. You need to get to another position. That's the softball field. To get from your school to the softball field, you need to change your position. To change your position, you have to be in motion.

**Motion** is a change in position. Any object that changes its position is in motion. The object can be a ball, a spaceship, or even you.

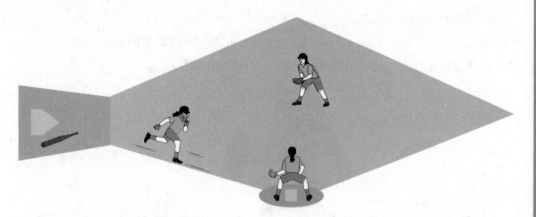

You are in motion hundreds of times each day. You stand up. You sit down. You walk from one room to another. You run from home plate to first base.

What causes these motions? Forces! A **force** is a push or a pull. A force can change the position of an object. A force can cause an object to move.

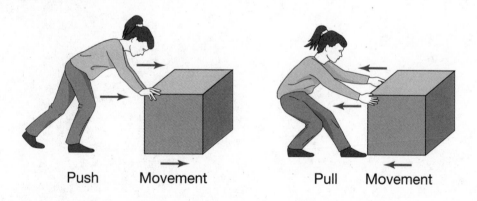

Push    Movement        Pull    Movement

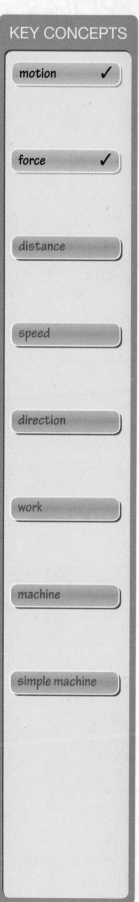

KEY CONCEPTS

motion ✓

force ✓

distance

speed

direction

work

machine

simple machine

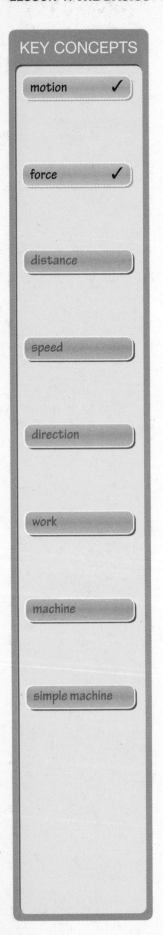

**KEY CONCEPTS**

motion ✓

force ✓

distance

speed

direction

work

machine

simple machine

You can also use a push to move yourself. Here's how you get up from a chair. Your feet push off from the floor. Your hands push off from the sides of the chair. These pushing forces change the position of your body. They put your body in motion.

Every time you take a step, your feet push on the ground. The backward push of your feet moves you forward.

How do you get your body to move forward when you are on rollerblades? You use a foot to push backward on the sidewalk. That backward force makes the skates roll forward.

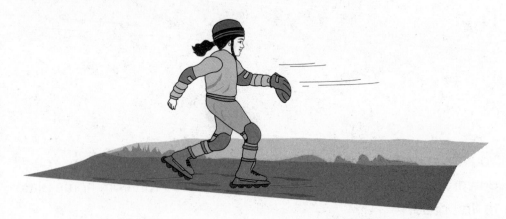

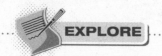

Make a log of the forces you use today. In the first column, classify the force as either a push or a pull. In the second column, name the object that received the force. In the third column, describe the effect the force had on the position of the object.

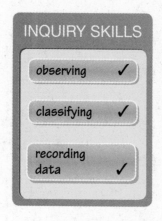

| Force | Object | Change of Position and Effect |
|---|---|---|
| Push | Pencil | I pushed my pencil across my paper to leave a mark. |
|  |  |  |
|  |  |  |
|  |  |  |
|  |  |  |
|  |  |  |

# LESSON 2: BUILDING ON THE BASICS

## KEY CONCEPTS

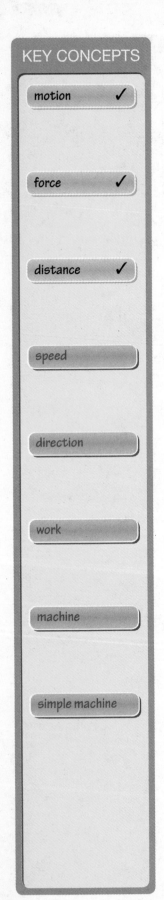

motion ✓

force ✓

distance ✓

speed

direction

work

machine

simple machine

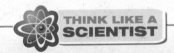

**THINK LIKE A SCIENTIST**

You walk out of school. Your watch reads 3:20. Now you have only 10 minutes to get to softball practice on time.

"I have a chance to make it on my rollerblades," you say to yourself.

You put on your skates. With all your might, you push off from the pavement. Swish. The skates and you spring into motion.

But will you get to practice on time? You get a bright idea.

"To answer the question, I need to know the distance to the field and the speed I will travel."

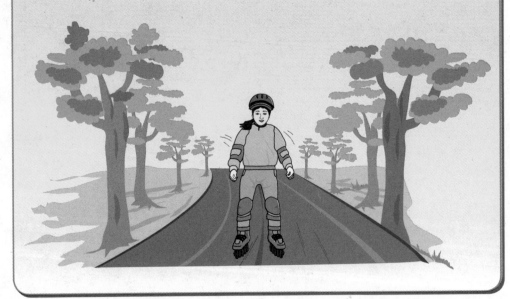

## Describing Motion

You know that force causes motion. Motion gets an object from one place to another. The space between the two places, and how far an object has moved, is called **distance**.

How long will it take you to travel the distance between your school and the field? That depends on how fast you skate. If you go fast, the trip will be short. If you go more slowly, the trip will be longer.

You will move faster if you push off with more force. That's why you push off with all your might. You want to put a large force on your skates.

## Speed

How fast an object moves is called **speed**. Speed is a measurement. It tells how fast or slowly an object moves across a distance.

You are a pitcher on your softball team. You throw the ball with as much speed as you can. What will make the ball go fast? The force you give to the ball.

If you swing your arm with great force, the ball will get to the batter quickly. It will travel the distance between you and the batter in a very short time. The ball's speed will be fast.

If you swing your arm with less force, the ball will take longer to travel between you and the batter. Its speed will be slower.

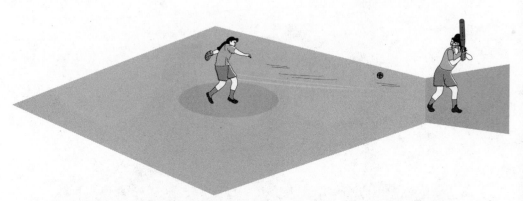

The pitcher pushes the ball forward. The stronger the force, the faster the ball will travel.

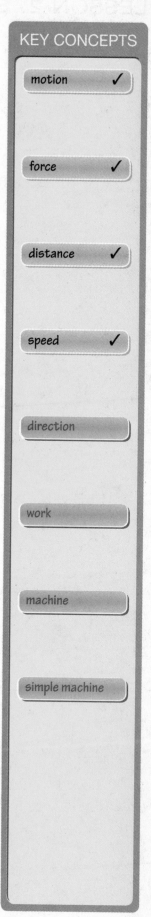

KEY CONCEPTS

motion ✓

force ✓

distance ✓

speed ✓

direction

work

machine

simple machine

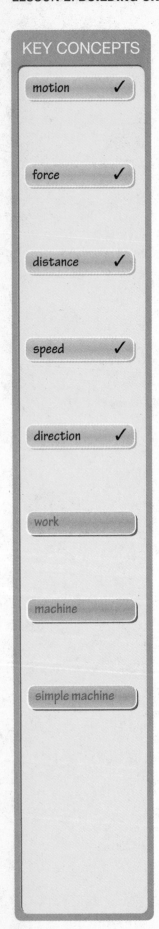

KEY CONCEPTS

motion ✓

force ✓

distance ✓

speed ✓

direction ✓

work

machine

simple machine

# Direction

You are on a moving object when you are skating. You and the skates are in motion. You need to control this motion to get to the softball field. You need to travel along a certain path. At times, the path may be straight. At other times, you may need to turn corners. The path you take as you move is your **direction**.

How do you change directions? You change the direction of the forces on the skates. If you want to go straight ahead, you push straight behind. If you want to go right, you push to the left. If you want to go left, you push to the right. The skates go in the opposite direction of your push. This is true of the movement of all objects.

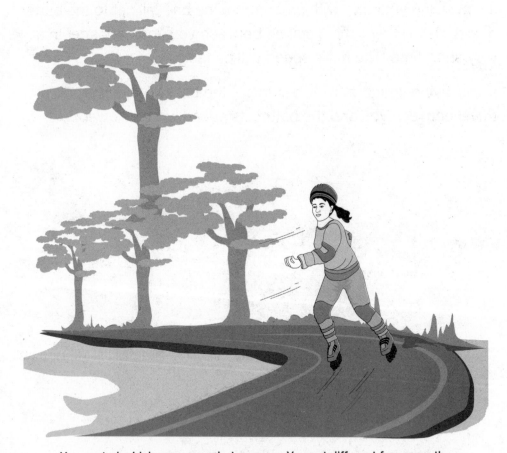

You control which way your skates move. You put different forces on the skates to make them move to the left, to the right, or straight ahead.

 **EXPLORE**

Change the speed and direction of a ball. Use different kinds of force. Observe the ball's motion. Make the ball move quickly, and then slowly. Make the ball move to the left and then to the right. Record your findings in the chart. In the second column, describe the force you used. In the third column, describe the motion of the ball.

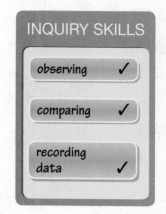

|  | Kind of Force Used | Motion of the Ball |
|---|---|---|
| **Changing Speed** |  |  |
|  |  |  |
| **Changing Direction** |  |  |
|  |  |  |

# LESSON 3: **BEYOND THE BASICS**

## KEY CONCEPTS

motion ✓

force ✓

distance ✓

speed ✓

direction ✓

work ✓

machine

simple machine

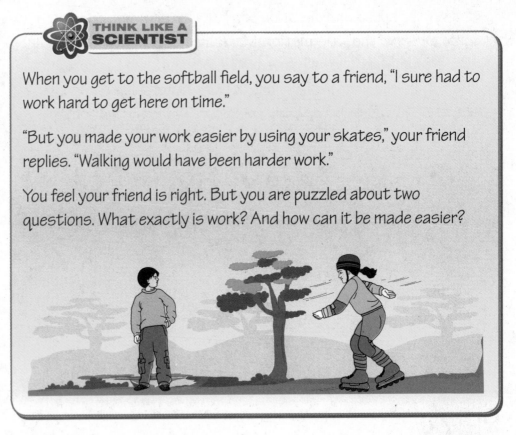

**THINK LIKE A SCIENTIST**

When you get to the softball field, you say to a friend, "I sure had to work hard to get here on time."

"But you made your work easier by using your skates," your friend replies. "Walking would have been harder work."

You feel your friend is right. But you are puzzled about two questions. What exactly is work? And how can it be made easier?

## Work and Machines

When you use a force to move an object a distance, you do **work**. You do work when you push your skates from your school to the softball field. You are using a force on the skates to move them a distance.

The boy in the picture is doing the same thing. Only he is pushing on the ground to get to the softball field. That's what he does every time he takes a step. Here's the difference. It's harder for the boy to walk to the field than it is for you to glide to it.

Your work is easier because you are using machines. The machines you are using are your skates.

# Machines

Your trip to the softball field was work. You used your skates to make the work easier. Skates are machines. A **machine** makes work easier. The machine does not lessen the amount of work. It lessens the amount of force needed to do the work.

Take a look at the drawings below. They show two ways to raise a box to a platform. Which way is easier? Pushing the box up the ramp is easier. A ramp is a machine that makes work easier. It takes less force to move the box up the ramp than to lift it straight up.

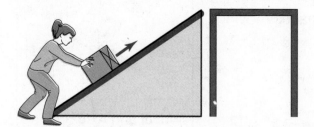 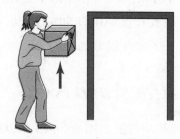

A **simple machine** is a tool that makes it easier to move an object. A simple machine has few or no moving parts. The inclined plane, lever, pulley, wedge, and wheel and axle are five kinds of simple machines.

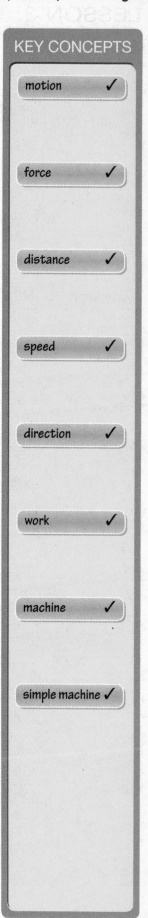

KEY CONCEPTS

| motion | ✓ |
| force | ✓ |
| distance | ✓ |
| speed | ✓ |
| direction | ✓ |
| work | ✓ |
| machine | ✓ |
| simple machine | ✓ |

Here are pictures of five simple machines. Each makes work easier.

# Lever

A lever is a bar that rests on a point. If you push down on one side of the lever, the other side moves up. A lever can help you lift something heavy.

# Inclined Plane

An inclined plane is a slanted surface, or a ramp. An inclined plane makes moving an object upward easier.

# Wheel and Axle

A wheel and axle is made up of a connected large and small wheel. The small wheel is the axle. Turning the larger wheel makes it easier to get the axle to turn. A screwdriver is a wheel and axle. It's easier to turn the handle, the wheel, than the thin rod, the axle.

# Wedge

A wedge is made up of one or more inclined planes. A wedge can help you pry an object apart.

# Pulley

A pulley is made up of a rope or chain around one or more wheels. You can use a pulley to lift heavy weights.

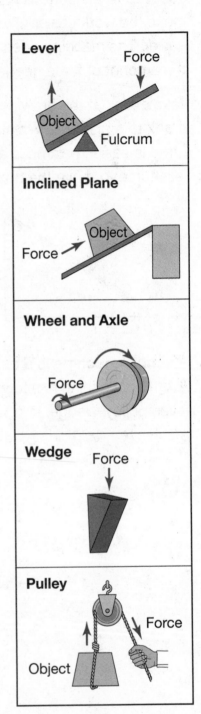

**Lever**
Force
Object
Fulcrum

**Inclined Plane**
Object
Force

**Wheel and Axle**
Force

**Wedge**
Force

**Pulley**
Force
Object

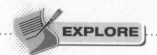 **EXPLORE**

Many everyday objects are machines. Look at tools that you use to move objects. Write the name of the tool in the box that tells what kind of machine it is. Then draw a picture of each tool.

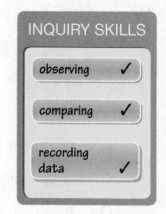

| Kind of Machine | Picture |
|---|---|
| Lever | |
| Inclined Plane | |
| Wedge | |
| Wheel and Axle | |
| Pulley | |

**INQUIRY SKILLS**

- observing ✓
- comparing ✓
- recording data ✓

# PUTTING IT ALL TOGETHER

**You are now ready to show you understand the key concepts covered in this topic. Read each question. Circle the letter of the best answer.**

1.  You use a pulling force to

    A.  skate.

    B.  throw a baseball.

    C.  play a piano.

    D.  open a refrigerator door.

2.  An object in motion is

    A.  always moving upward.

    B.  changing its position.

    C.  moving from left to right.

    D.  moving very quickly.

3.  A force in one direction will cause

    A.  motion in the opposite direction.

    B.  motion in the same direction.

    C.  no motion.

    D.  motion to start and stop.

4.  Speed is a measure of

    A.  how much force was put on an object.

    B.  the path a moving object takes.

    C.  how fast an object moves.

    D.  how long an object moves.

5.  Work is done when

    A.  a force moves an object.

    B.  an object changes direction.

    C.  an object changes speed.

    D.  a force is put on an object.

6.  A machine always makes

    A.  a moving object gain speed.

    B.  an object stop moving.

    C.  a moving object change direction.

    D.  work easier.

**7.** Which of the following is a wedge?

    **A.** diving board

    **B.** knife

    **C.** doorknob

    **D.** baseball bat

**8.** A doorknob is an example of a

    **A.** pulley.

    **B.** wedge.

    **C.** wheel and axle.

    **D.** lever.

**9.** A machine helps you

    **A.** do less work.

    **B.** use more motion to do work.

    **C.** do work faster.

    **D.** use less force to do work.

**10.** Which is an example of work?

    **A.** holding a pencil

    **B.** picking up an apple

    **C.** talking to a friend

    **D.** watching a movie

# Physical Properties of Matter

. . . . . . . . . . . . . . . . . . . . . . . . . . . . . . . . . . . . . . . . . . . . . .

## LESSON 1: THE BASICS

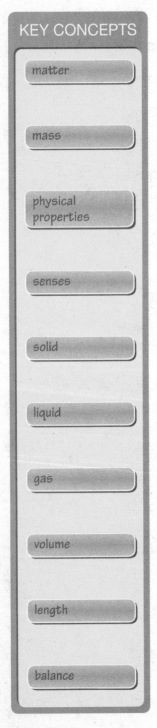

### KEY CONCEPTS

- matter
- mass
- physical properties
- senses
- solid
- liquid
- gas
- volume
- length
- balance

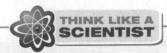

**THINK LIKE A SCIENTIST**

You and your family are visiting Crater of Diamonds State Park in Arkansas. In this park, visitors are allowed to dig for diamonds. Best of all, you may keep any diamonds you find!

You push your shovel into the ground. You look closely at the soil. Nothing! You dig up another shovelful of soil. Suddenly, you see two pebbles. What are they?

You bring the pebbles to a park ranger. "Could these be diamonds?" you ask.

"Might be. Might not be. Could be quartz," the ranger replies.

"What's quartz?" you say.

"An ordinary kind of rock," says the ranger.

Are the pebbles quartz? Diamonds? Or one of each? "What do I need to know to answer the questions?" you wonder.

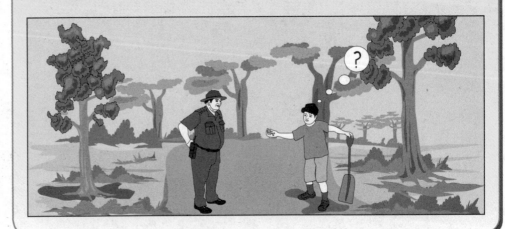

# Observing Matter

The pebbles you found are kinds of **matter**. Matter is anything that has mass and takes up space. **Mass** is the "stuff" in an object. Objects with more mass weigh more than objects with less mass. Matter is all around you. Your shovel and the soil are made of matter. So are you. So are the mysterious pebbles you dug up.

How can you find out if the pebbles are diamonds, quartz, or one of each? You can be a scientific detective. You can look for clues to what the pebbles are. Some of those clues are the pebbles' physical properties.

A **physical property** is something you can observe about an object. Color is a physical property. Shape is a physical property. The size and weight of an object are physical properties. Hardness is a physical property. The temperature at which an object melts or freezes is a physical property.

What are some physical properties of this shell and this pebble?

An object's physical properties can help you figure out what it is. That's because each kind of matter has its own set of physical properties.

The seashell shown above is hard. The pebbles you found on your diamond hunt are harder. The shell and pebbles are also different colors, sizes, and shapes. Each has a different set of physical properties. They are different kinds of matter.

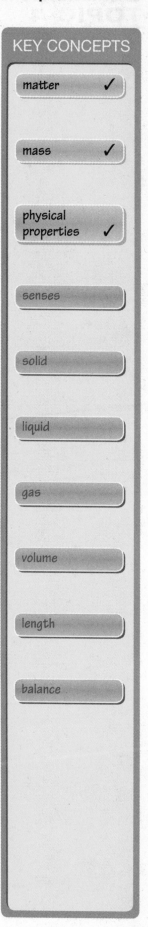

KEY CONCEPTS

matter ✓

mass ✓

physical properties ✓

senses

solid

liquid

gas

volume

length

balance

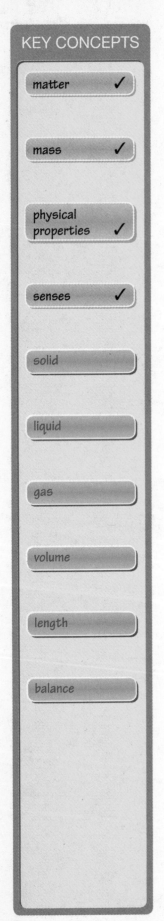

KEY CONCEPTS

matter ✓

mass ✓

physical properties ✓

senses ✓

solid

liquid

gas

volume

length

balance

You use your **senses** to observe the physical properties of an object. Your five senses are sight, hearing, smell, taste, and touch.

Using your sense of sight, you observe that your mysterious pebbles are white. You see that they are about the size of a pea.

Your sight and touch tell you that they are smooth. Your sense of touch also tells you that the pebbles are very hard.

You record your observations in a notebook. Each property you write down brings you a step closer to figuring out what the pebbles are.

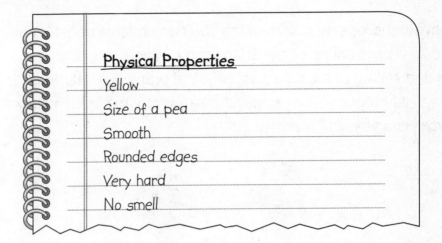

Physical Properties
Yellow
Size of a pea
Smooth
Rounded edges
Very hard
No smell

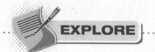

Choose two objects. Write their names above each column. Use your senses to observe the physical properties of each object. Record your observations in the table. **NOTE: DO NOT TASTE AN UNKNOWN OBJECT OR ONE THAT COULD HARM YOU.** You may taste foods sold in a market or grocery.

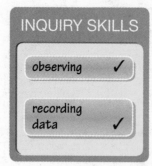

INQUIRY SKILLS

observing ✓

recording data ✓

|  | Object 1 | Object 2 |
|---|---|---|
| What You See |  |  |
| What You Hear |  |  |
| What You Smell |  |  |
| What You Taste |  |  |
| What You Feel |  |  |

# LESSON 2: BUILDING ON THE BASICS

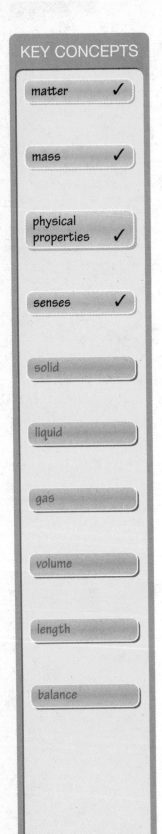

KEY CONCEPTS

- matter ✓
- mass ✓
- physical properties ✓
- senses ✓
- solid
- liquid
- gas
- volume
- length
- balance

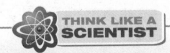

**THINK LIKE A SCIENTIST**

You have used your senses to observe some of the physical properties of the mysterious pebbles. One thing is clear. The pebbles are solids. But all pebbles are solids. Diamonds are solids. So is a piece of quartz.

You ask yourself, "If all pebbles are solids, how can I figure out if these pebbles are diamonds, or quartz, or one of each?" The answer is in their properties.

Solids can change into liquids. Liquids can even change into gases. But different kinds of solids change into liquids at different temperatures. The temperature at which a solid turns into a liquid is one of its physical properties.

You think, "If I can find the temperature where the pebbles turn into liquids, I might have a clue to what they are. But first, I should understand the science of solids, liquids, and gases."

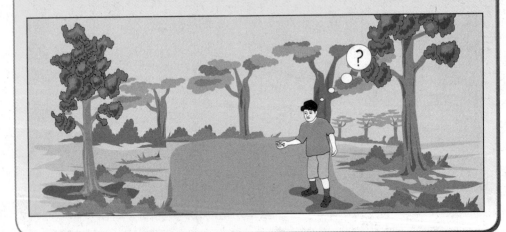

## States of Matter

How are a solid, a liquid, and a gas different?

All matter is made up of tiny pieces. You cannot see these pieces, but they are there. Diamonds and quartz are made up of such pieces.

If you could see the smallest pieces of matter, you would observe them moving. In some matter, the particles move very slowly. In other kinds of matter, the particles move quickly.

The particles that make up matter are arranged differently, too. In some matter, the particles are packed close together. In other matter, the particles are spread far apart.

When you heat up a solid, like a pebble, the pieces in it move faster. They also move apart. What happens if the pieces move fast enough and far enough apart? The solid will turn into a liquid. This is called a change of state.

Matter comes in three different states. These are solids, liquids, and gases. Let's explore the properties of each of these states.

## Solids

The particles of a **solid** move very slowly. They are packed close together. This gives the solid a definite shape.

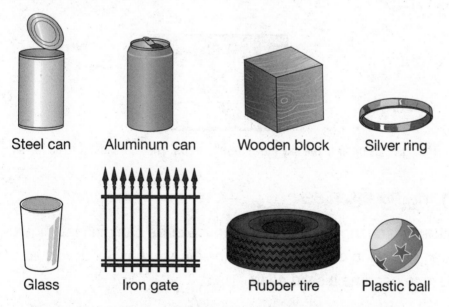

| Steel can | Aluminum can | Wooden block | Silver ring |

| Glass | Iron gate | Rubber tire | Plastic ball |

The particles that make up these solids are tightly packed. This makes the solids keep their shape and take up a certain amount of space.

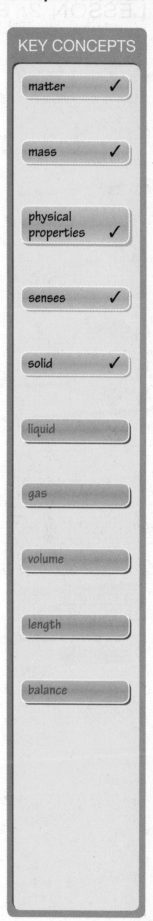

KEY CONCEPTS

matter ✓

mass ✓

physical properties ✓

senses ✓

solid ✓

liquid

gas

volume

length

balance

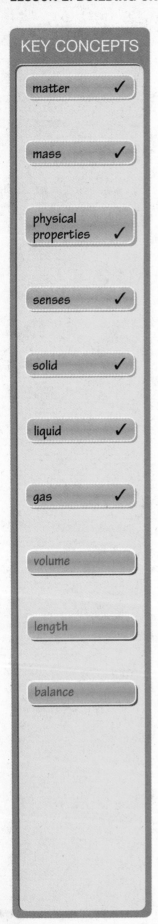

matter ✓

mass ✓

physical properties ✓

senses ✓

solid ✓

liquid ✓

gas ✓

volume

length

balance

## Liquids

The particles of a **liquid** can move past one another. They are loosely packed. So the liquid does not have a definite shape.

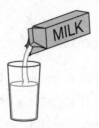

MILK

Milk is a liquid. The milk in the carton takes the shape of the carton. The milk in the glass takes the shape of the glass. Even though the shape of the liquid changes, the amount of space it takes up stays the same.

## Gases

The particles of a **gas** move very quickly. They are not packed together. They can move around freely. The particles that make up a gas can spread out in all directions. So the amount of space a gas takes up can change.

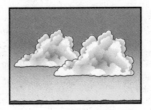

The particles of air in the sky move around freely. They spread out to fill the sky.

## Changing States

Matter can change its state. A solid ice cube can melt into liquid water. The puddle can move into the air as a gas. Or the liquid can freeze to become a solid again.

 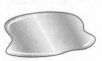

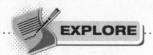 **EXPLORE**

Complete the three-column chart. Describe each state of matter. Then give examples of each.

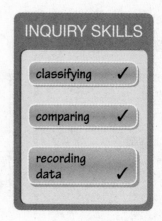

INQUIRY SKILLS

classifying ✓

comparing ✓

recording data ✓

| Solids | Liquids | Gases |
|---|---|---|
| Description: | Description: | Description: |
| Examples: | Examples: | Examples: |

# LESSON 3: **BEYOND THE BASICS**

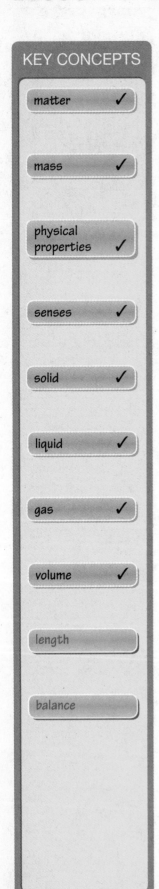

KEY CONCEPTS

| | |
|---|---|
| matter | ✓ |
| mass | ✓ |
| physical properties | ✓ |
| senses | ✓ |
| solid | ✓ |
| liquid | ✓ |
| gas | ✓ |
| volume | ✓ |
| length | |
| balance | |

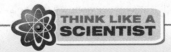

**THINK LIKE A SCIENTIST**

You know that different solids melt at different temperatures. And you know that different solids have different hardnesses. So now it's time to measure the temperature at which your pebbles melt. And it's also time to measure their hardness.

You ask yourself, "At what temperature do diamonds and quartz melt? What is their hardness? And how do I measure their hardness, anyway?"

To find the answers, you have to do some research.

You go to your library or to the Internet and read about the properties of diamonds and quartz. You also read about hardness and how to measure it.

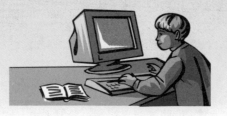

## Measuring Matter

After you complete your research, this is what you have found about the melting temperature and hardness of diamonds and quartz.

| Object | Temperature at Which It Melts | Hardness |
|---|---|---|
| Diamond | 4440°C | 10 |
| Quartz | 1713°C | 7 |

You can measure temperature and hardness. Here are some other physical properties of matter you can measure.

## Volume

**Volume** is the amount of space that an object takes up.

A measuring cup is one tool used to measure the volume of a liquid. You pour the liquid into the cup. Then you read the numbered units on its side.

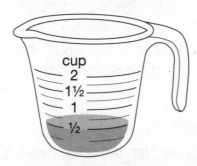

What is the volume of the liquid
in this measuring cup?

## Length

**Length** is the distance from one place to another.

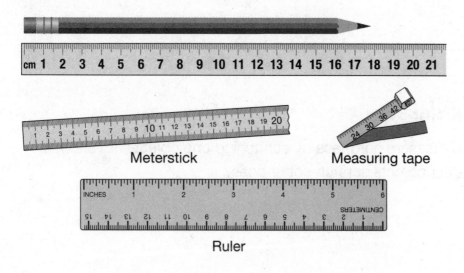

Meterstick                    Measuring tape

Ruler

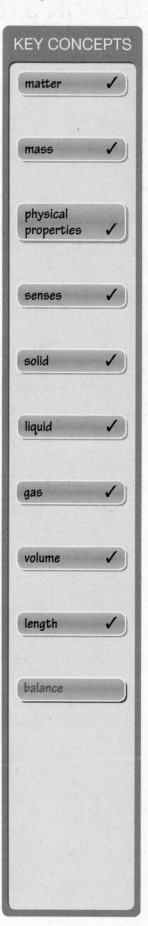

KEY CONCEPTS

matter ✓

mass ✓

physical properties ✓

senses ✓

solid ✓

liquid ✓

gas ✓

volume ✓

length ✓

balance

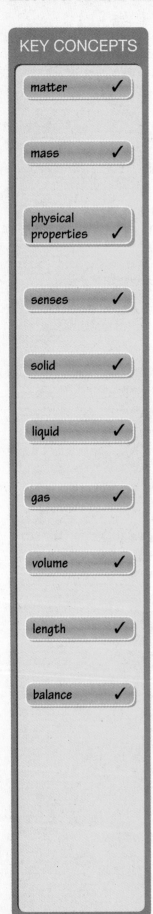

KEY CONCEPTS

matter ✓

mass ✓

physical properties ✓

senses ✓

solid ✓

liquid ✓

gas ✓

volume ✓

length ✓

balance ✓

# Mass

Mass is the amount of matter in an object. You can use a **balance** to measure mass.

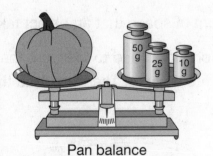

Pan balance

You would use a balance to find the mass of an object.

# Temperature

You measure temperature with a thermometer. Other instruments are used to measure very high temperatures.

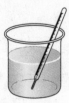

A thermometer is used to measure temperatures that are not too high or too low.

# Hardness

You measure hardness by scratching one object with another. Harder objects scratch softer ones.

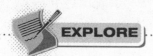

**EXPLORE**

Hardness is measured from 1 to 10. Ten is hardest. One is softest. Harder objects scratch softer ones. Go back and look at what you discovered about the hardness and melting temperature of diamonds and quartz. Remember, you found two pebbles. Are they both diamonds? Both quartz? You can solve the mystery by examining the physical properties described in the chart. Write your conclusions in the chart.

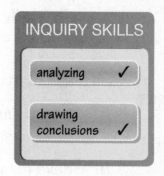

INQUIRY SKILLS

analyzing ✓

drawing conclusions ✓

| Pebble 1 | Pebble 2 |
|---|---|
| Scratches object with a hardness of 6.<br><br>Does not scratch object with a hardness of 8.<br><br>Melts at a temperature between 1700°C and 1750°C.<br><br>Solid 1 is _____ | Scratches all objects with a hardness of 1–9.<br><br>Is still solid at 4000°C.<br><br>Solid 2 is _____ |

# PUTTING IT ALL TOGETHER

**You are now ready to show you understand the key concepts covered in this topic. Read each question. Circle the letter of the best answer.**

1. All types of matter

   A. take up space and have a definite shape.

   B. have mass and taste.

   C. take up space and have mass.

   D. have a definite size and shape.

2. All solids, liquids, and gases are made of particles that

   A. are packed close together.

   B. are tightly packed.

   C. slide past one another.

   D. are always moving.

3. When an ice cube melts, it changes from

   A. a solid to a liquid.

   B. a liquid to a gas.

   C. a solid to a gas.

   D. a gas to a solid.

4. Which of the following is NOT a tool used to measure matter?

   A. ruler

   B. balance

   C. measuring cup

   D. hand lens

5. Which physical property can you observe with your sense of touch?

   A. height

   B. roughness

   C. sourness

   D. brightness

6. How are gases and liquids alike?

   A. They do not have a definite shape.

   B. They do not have a definite mass.

   C. They are not made up of particles.

   D. They do not have physical properties.

7. Which of the following is a group of solids?

    A. rain, bathtub, umbrella

    B. snow, shovel, boots

    C. milk, apple, ice cube

    D. glove, shoe, cloud

8. If a solid has a hardness of 5, it will scratch another solid with a hardness of

    A. 4.

    B. 6.

    C. 7.

    D. 8.

9. Which of the following is a tool used to measure length?

    A. a meterstick

    B. a measuring cup

    C. a thermometer

    D. a balance

10. Which of the following has the greatest mass?

    A. dime

    B. pencil

    C. computer

    D. cup

# Energy Forms and Changes

## LESSON 1: **THE BASICS**

### KEY CONCEPTS

- energy
- potential energy
- kinetic energy
- heat energy
- chemical energy
- mechanical energy
- electrical energy
- thermal energy

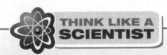

**THINK LIKE A SCIENTIST**

At last! You're on your camping trip. You and your family have found a spot for your tent.

You begin to help set up the tent. Then, a few questions pop into your mind. How will you keep warm during the chilly nights? How will you keep animals from eating the food you brought along in your backpack?

You are not sure of the answers. But you have an idea they have something to do with energy. Then another question pops into your mind. What is energy, anyway?

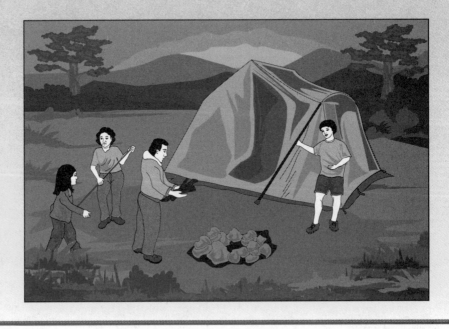

# What Is Energy?

**Energy** is the ability to make things change. What kinds of change?

Energy can change something from cool to warm. It can keep you warm on a cool night. It can melt an ice cube.

Energy can move things, too. Energy can raise a tent. It can clear a boulder from a campsite.

Energy can help you turn a pile of wood into a campfire. And it can turn on a flashlight.

You and your family set up camp. You need to find a safe place to store your backpack full of food. You do not want animals to eat the food. You spot a tall tree nearby. If you could string the backpack over one of the branches, the food might be safe. But the tree is too hard to climb. How are you going to get the backpack up there?

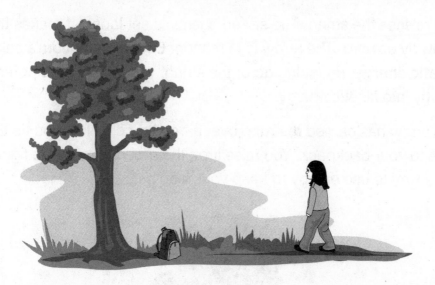

You get a bright idea. Maybe you can use the bow and arrow you brought with you to help get the backpack into the tree. You tie a rope to the arrow. You place the arrow in the bow. Then you pull back the string of the bow. When you pull back the string, you store energy in the bow.

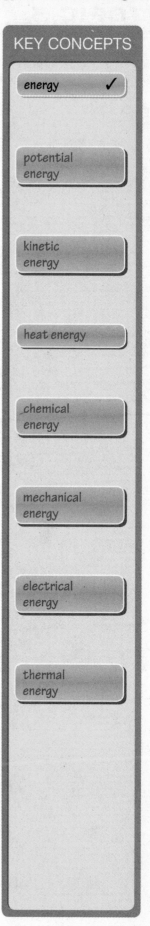

KEY CONCEPTS

energy  ✓

potential energy

kinetic energy

heat energy

chemical energy

mechanical energy

electrical energy

thermal energy

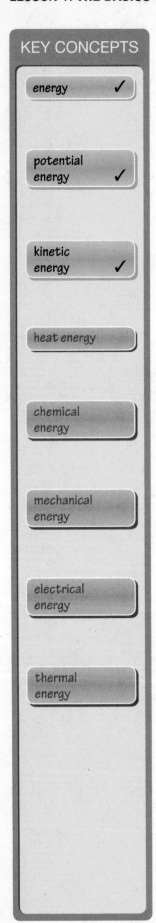

KEY CONCEPTS

energy ✓

potential energy ✓

kinetic energy ✓

heat energy

chemical energy

mechanical energy

electrical energy

thermal energy

Stored energy is **potential energy**. It's saved energy. It's like coins you have saved in a drawer. You aren't using the money yet. But you can.

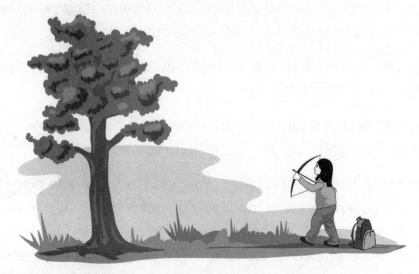

The stretched bow has potential energy.

You release the string. The stored energy is set loose. It makes the arrow fly upward. The arrow is in motion. Energy of motion is called **kinetic energy**. By letting go of the string, you've changed potential energy into kinetic energy.

The arrow has carried the rope over a tree branch. Now you tie the rope to your backpack. You raise it off the ground. You have figured out a way to use energy to keep your food safe.

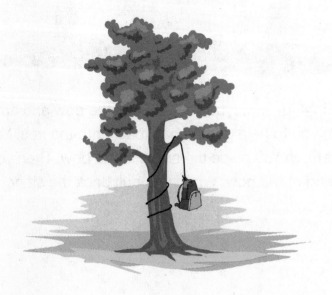

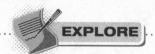 **EXPLORE**

Look at the pictures below. Tell whether each picture shows potential or kinetic energy. Then tell how you know. Remember to ask yourself if the energy is stored (potential) or moving (kinetic).

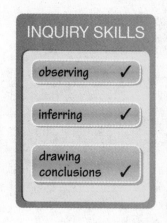

| KINETIC AND POTENTIAL ENERGY | | |
|---|---|---|
| What I See | Type of Energy | How I Know |
|  |  |  |
|  |  |  |
|  |  |  |
|  |  |  |

# LESSON 2: BUILDING ON THE BASICS

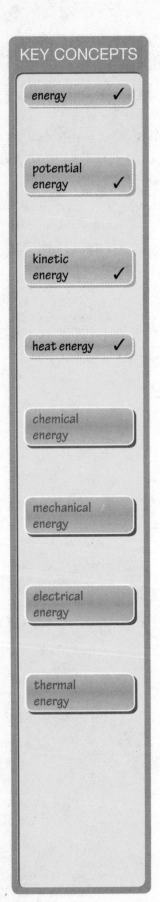

## KEY CONCEPTS

- energy ✓
- potential energy ✓
- kinetic energy ✓
- heat energy ✓
- chemical energy
- mechanical energy
- electrical energy
- thermal energy

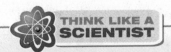

**THINK LIKE A SCIENTIST**

You have helped set up your family's tent. And you have found a way to keep your food safe from animals. Now you can sit down to rest.

You sit on a rock and watch the sun setting. A cool breeze begins to blow. Your hands start to feel cold. You shiver. You think again about getting warm. It makes you wonder. "What form of energy makes me get warm?"

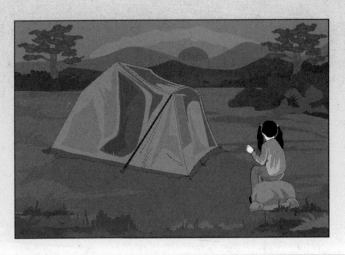

## Forms of Energy

Your father said he would make hot soup for supper. If you put your cool hands on the warm bowl, your hands will warm up. Heat will move from the bowl to your hands. Heat always moves from warmer objects to cooler ones. **Heat energy** is what makes your hands get warm.

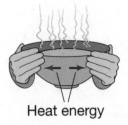

Heat energy

Heat energy is one form of energy. Energy comes in other forms, too. **Chemical energy** is energy stored inside a material, such as wood.

Objects in motion have mechanical energy. You have mechanical energy when you run. **Mechanical energy** is energy of motion. Mechanical energy is a kind of kinetic energy. Wind has mechanical energy. Flowing water has it, too.

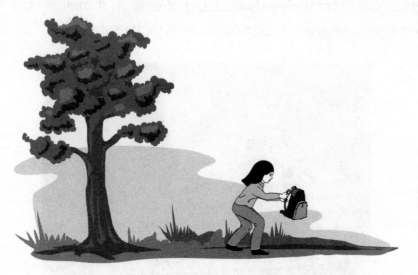

You use mechanical energy when you lift a backpack.

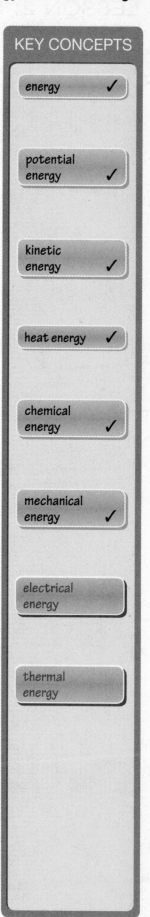

KEY CONCEPTS

| energy | ✓ |
| potential energy | ✓ |
| kinetic energy | ✓ |
| heat energy | ✓ |
| chemical energy | ✓ |
| mechanical energy | ✓ |
| electrical energy | |
| thermal energy | |

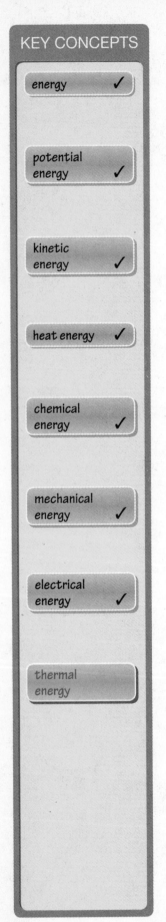

KEY CONCEPTS

- energy ✓
- potential energy ✓
- kinetic energy ✓
- heat energy ✓
- chemical energy ✓
- mechanical energy ✓
- electrical energy ✓
- thermal energy

You've probably had a lot of experience with **electrical energy**. Most electrical energy comes from power plants. It can also come from batteries.

You can find a battery near the engine in a car. It helps get the car started. You can find batteries in flashlights, too.

Electrical energy is also found in nature as lightning!

Electrical energy is a very useful form of energy. It makes your home's lights, television, computer, and refrigerator work.

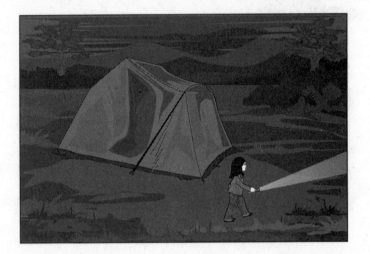

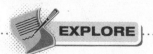 **EXPLORE**

Choose four different machines that use electricity. They can be in your school or home. Tell what kind of energy each machine produces. For example, a clothes dryer produces heat energy. Remember that forms of energy include heat, light, and motion. List at least one machine for each form of energy.

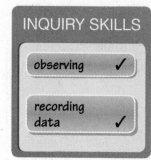

INQUIRY SKILLS

observing ✓

recording data ✓

| FORMS OF ENERGY | |
|---|---|
| Machine | Form of Energy |
| Clothes dryer | Heat energy |
| | |
| | |
| | |
| | |

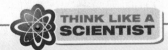

**THINK LIKE A SCIENTIST**

By now the sun has set. The evening is getting cold. You gather twigs and logs. You pile them up. Your mother strikes a match to start a campfire. Before long, the wood is blazing.

Your family has gathered around. The fire warms everyone. You are comfortable. You can relax. You have time to think.

"Where is the energy of the fire coming from?" you wonder. "Could it have been inside the wood all along?"

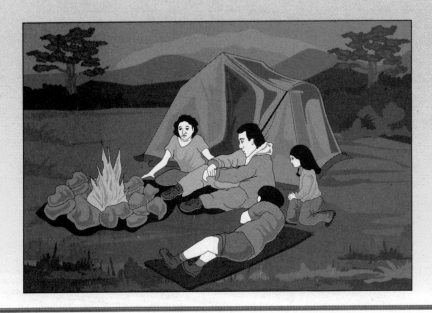

## Energy Changes Form

Twigs and logs are not hot. They don't seem to hold energy. But they produce heat when they burn. Where did the heat come from?

When you burn a log, you let loose chemical energy that was stored in the wood. The chemical energy turns into two other kinds of energy—light energy and heat energy. That's why you see flames and feel heat when wood burns. Heat energy is also called **thermal energy**.

The material on the head of a match holds chemical energy, too. Striking the match on a rough surface heats the material up. It heats up just enough to start burning. So striking a match also turns chemical energy into light energy and thermal energy.

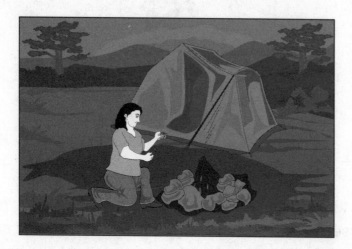

Batteries also hold chemical energy. When you switch on a flashlight, the chemical energy changes into electrical energy. Then the electrical energy is changed into light energy by the lightbulb. Some of the electrical energy changes into heat energy, too. The bulb gets warm.

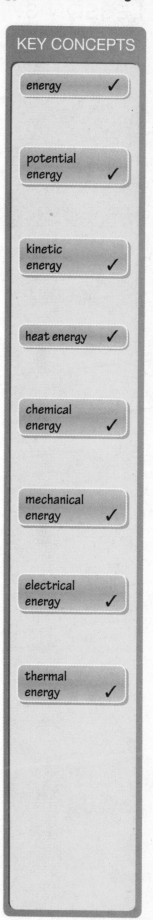

KEY CONCEPTS

energy ✓

potential energy ✓

kinetic energy ✓

heat energy ✓

chemical energy ✓

mechanical energy ✓

electrical energy ✓

thermal energy ✓

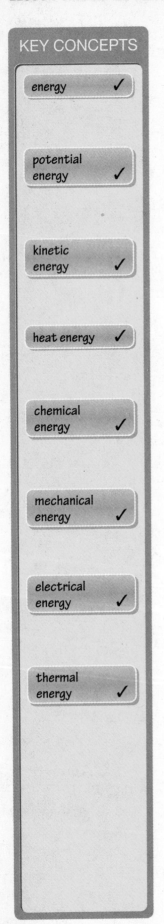

KEY CONCEPTS

energy ✓

potential energy ✓

kinetic energy ✓

heat energy ✓

chemical energy ✓

mechanical energy ✓

electrical energy ✓

thermal energy ✓

Back at home you use many machines that change energy from one form to another. In a toaster, electrical energy is mostly turned into heat energy.

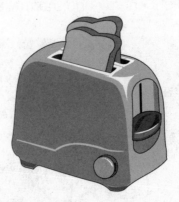

A blender turns electrical energy into mechanical energy. Your television set turns electrical energy into light energy and sound energy. A lightbulb turns electrical energy into light and heat energy.

Turn on a gas stove, and you change chemical energy into heat and light energy. Eat a banana and run around the block. Inside your body, you have changed some of the chemical energy in the banana to the energy of motion—your running legs.

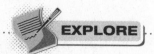

Make a list of what you do on an ordinary day. The list might include homework, play, travel, chores, or other activities. Choose four activities. Write them in the boxes at the left. Then in the boxes at the right tell what kinds of energy changes happened during each activity.

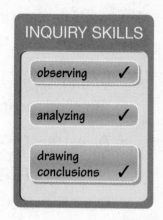

| ENERGY CHANGES FORM | |
| --- | --- |
| Activity | Energy Changes |
|  |  |
|  |  |
|  |  |
|  |  |

# PUTTING IT ALL TOGETHER

**You are now ready to show you understand the key concepts covered in this topic. Read each question. Circle the letter of the best answer.**

1. What happens if you put a cool metal spoon in warm water?

   A. The spoon gets cooler.

   B. The spoon gets warmer.

   C. The spoon stays the same temperature.

   D. The spoon dissolves.

2. Which is another name for stored energy?

   A. motion

   B. heat energy

   C. kinetic energy

   D. potential energy

3. When you switch on a lamp, you are converting

   A. electrical energy into light.

   B. heat energy into light.

   C. kinetic energy into motion.

   D. potential energy into sound.

4. Standing on top of a hill, you have

   A. only kinetic energy.

   B. both potential and kinetic energy.

   C. only potential energy.

   D. no energy.

5. Which is a true statement about energy?

   A. Energy cannot change form.

   B. Energy can change form.

   C. Energy has weight.

   D. There is only one form of energy.

6. Anna's mother used wood and matches to start a campfire. The campfire produces

   A. heat and light.

   B. only light.

   C. only heat.

   D. electricity.

7. What kind of energy does an apple hold?

   A. light

   B. chemical

   C. thermal

   D. mechanical

8. Which changes electrical energy into motion?

   A. a fan

   B. a lamp

   C. a flashlight

   D. a jet airplane

9. When you hit a ball with a bat, what kind of energy sends the ball flying?

   A. kinetic energy

   B. potential energy

   C. heat energy

   D. sound energy

10. Which statement about heat is true?

   A. Heat does not move.

   B. Heat is not energy.

   C. Heat moves from a warmer object to a cooler object.

   D. Heat moves from a cooler object to a warmer object.

# Adaptations and Change over Time

## LESSON 1: **THE BASICS**

KEY CONCEPTS

adaptation ✓

environment

climate

extinct

fossil

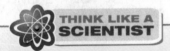

**THINK LIKE A SCIENTIST**

You are on a beach. A small crab runs over the sand. A sea star clings to a rock. Dune grasses grow in the sand behind you. You watch as fish wiggle in the waves that hit the beach. Farther out in the ocean, you see dolphins jump into the air and dive back into the sea. High above, seagulls squawk as they search for food. You wonder, what makes these living things suited to life in or near the water?

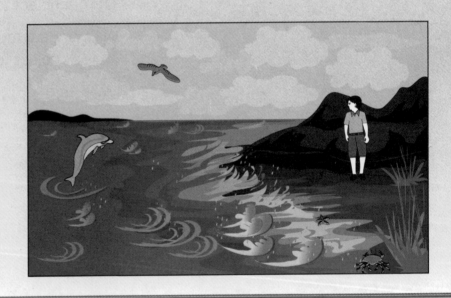

## Adaptations

For millions of years, animals and plants have lived in and near the sea. Many kinds have died out. But some have lived on. Those that have lived on have traits that have helped them survive. A trait can be a body part. It can also be a way of living. Traits that help a living thing to survive are called **adaptations**. Adaptations are passed from parents to their young. All the living things in the picture are adapted to the sea and seashore. What kinds of adaptations do they have?

A crab has five pairs of legs. Some of those legs are adapted for moving quickly over sand. Some are adapted to catch and hold food. The back legs of some crabs are adapted for swimming.

Look at the sea star. What keeps the waves from washing the animal off the rock? A sea star has sticky cups on the bottom of its body. They hold it firmly to the rock. That's its adaptation to a place washed by waves.

Fish and dolphins are also adapted to life in water. Both have body shapes that help them glide through water. Fish have fins and dolphins have flippers. They use the flippers and fins to swim. Fins and flippers are adaptations to life in water.

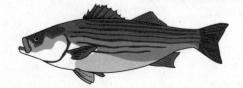 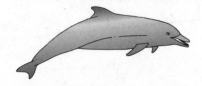

The underground stems of dune grasses are adapted to a sandy, windy place. They are long and hold on well to shifting sand. Without such stems, dune grasses would blow away and die.

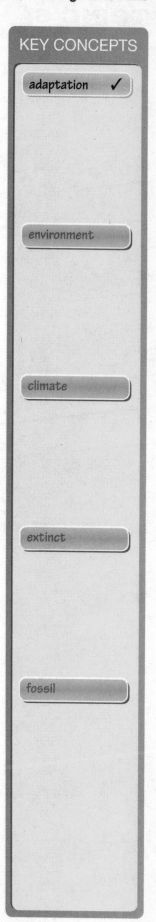

KEY CONCEPTS

adaptation ✓

environment

climate

extinct

fossil

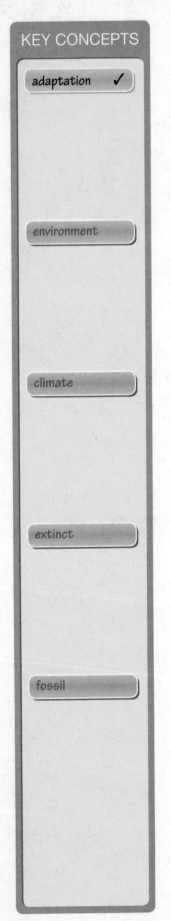

**KEY CONCEPTS**

adaptation ✓

environment

climate

extinct

fossil

Sea birds are adapted to a life above, on, or in the sea. Most sea birds have waterproof feathers. The feathers don't soak up water. Water-soaked birds would have a hard time flying.

Most sea birds have webbed feet. They use their webbed feet to swim.

Some sea birds that dive for fish have short wings. This allows them to dive faster and deeper. Other sea birds have sharp beaks to spear fish.

The wings of penguins are adapted for life in water. Penguins use their wings for swimming, not flying.

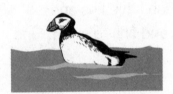 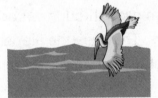 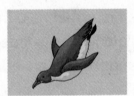

**EXPLORE**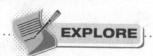

Look closely at each animal below, and name one adaptation of each. Then tell how you think the adaptation helps the animal meet its needs.

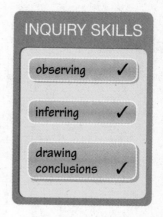

INQUIRY SKILLS

observing ✓

inferring ✓

drawing conclusions ✓

| MORE ADAPTATIONS | | |
|---|---|---|
| Animal | Adaptation | How I Think the Adaptation Helps the Animal |
| Sea Turtle | | |
| Clam | | |
| Shark | | |
| Stingray | | |
| Jellyfish | | |

## KEY CONCEPTS

adaptation ✓

environment ✓

climate ✓

extinct

fossil

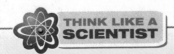 **THINK LIKE A SCIENTIST**

Imagine that you are back at the beach. But now it is *one thousand years* later! You look around. There are no grasses on the dunes. The air has become much colder. The waves beat much harder on the rocks. You wonder, how do changes in an environment affect the things that live there?

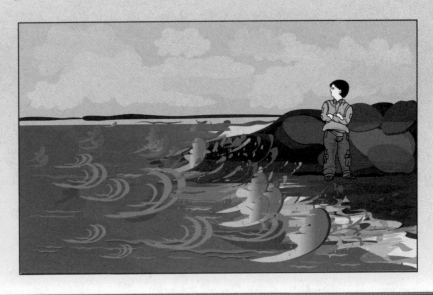

## Changing Environments

Everything that surrounds a living thing makes up its **environment**. Some parts of an environment are nonliving, or not alive. Air, water, waves, sand, and climate are nonliving parts of a beach environment.

**Climate** is the kind of weather a place usually gets over a long time. The time can be years. The climate of a desert is usually hot and dry. The climate of a beach can be cool and wet.

Other parts of an environment are living. Crabs, seagulls, grasses, fish, and dolphins are just a few of the living parts of an ocean and beach environment.

All of these living things are adapted to their environment. They have traits that help them survive there *now*. But these traits might not help them survive as the environment changes.

For example, the dune grasses might not survive if the climate becomes very dry. The crabs might not survive if the climate turns very cold. And gulls that eat the crabs might not survive if the crabs disappear. Sea stars might be swept away if the waves get too strong.

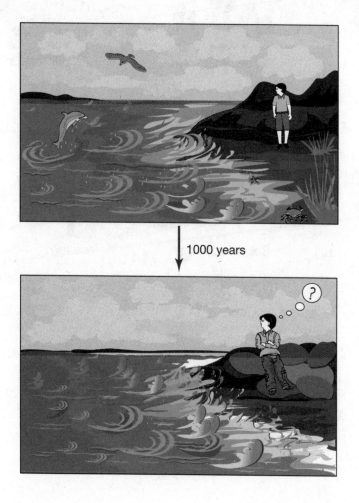

1000 years

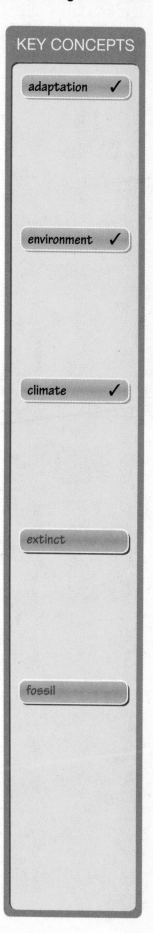

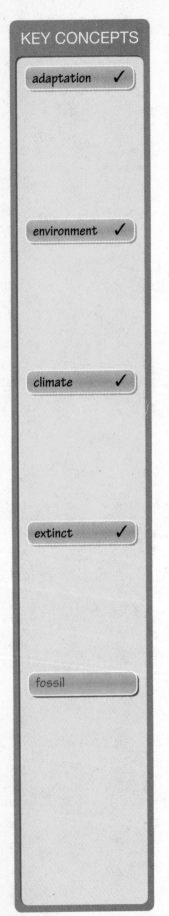

KEY CONCEPTS

adaptation ✓

environment ✓

climate ✓

extinct ✓

fossil

What happens if all of a kind of living thing die out? That kind of living thing becomes extinct. **Extinct** means gone forever. All the living things shown below are extinct.

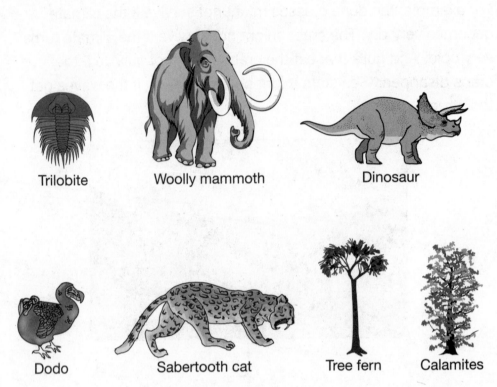

Trilobite          Woolly mammoth          Dinosaur

Dodo          Sabertooth cat          Tree fern          Calamites

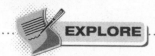

**EXPLORE**

This chart lists some living things that could soon become extinct.
It also gives the reason. Use the chart to answer the questions.

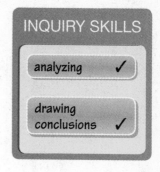

INQUIRY SKILLS

analyzing ✓

drawing conclusions ✓

| Kind of Living Thing | Some Reasons the Kind of Living Thing Is in Danger |
|---|---|
| Blue whale | • Illegal hunting<br>• Pollution |
| Loggerhead turtle | • Changing beaches<br>• Getting stuck in fishing nets |
| Atlantic salmon | • Too much fishing<br>• Disease |
| Elkhorn coral | • Warming ocean<br>• Pollution |
| White abalone | • Too much fishing<br>• Disease |
| Johnson's sea grass | • Loss of beaches<br>• Storms |

1. What is a danger to loggerhead turtles?

_____

2. Which two kinds of living thing are losing numbers to diseases?

_____

3. Which living thing is losing numbers because of storms?

_____

4. Which kind of living thing is in danger because the ocean
   is warming?

_____

5. Why is the number of blue whales getting smaller?

_____

# LESSON 3: **BEYOND THE BASICS**

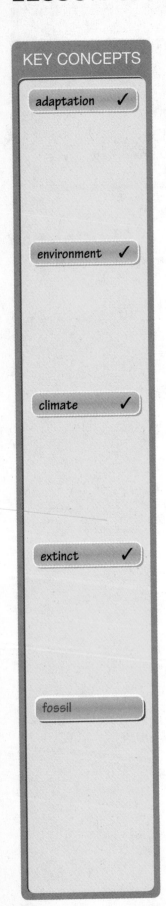

KEY CONCEPTS

adaptation ✓

environment ✓

climate ✓

extinct ✓

fossil

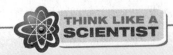

**THINK LIKE A SCIENTIST**

Imagine that you are once again at the beach. It is *one million years later!* You look around. The water is still there, but the dunes and beach are gone. In their place is a wall of rock filled with shells and fish bones. Many questions fill your head. What kinds of living things did these shells and bones belong to? How did they get into these rocks? What can they tell me about life here long, long ago?

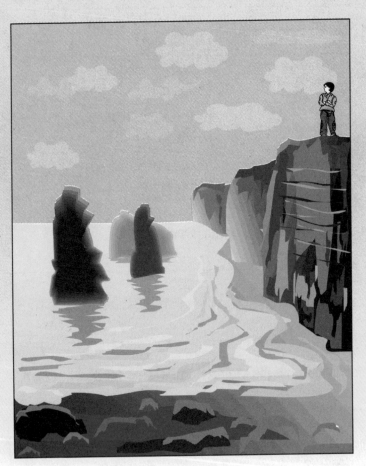

# Fossils

The shells and fish bones in the rocks are fossils. A **fossil** is any evidence or remains of an ancient living thing. Fossils are preserved in different ways. What kinds of ways?

Think back to the beach you first visited. The sand was soft and loose. Now it's a million years later. The sand is hard rock. How did the shells and bones get into the rock?

The remains of the fish and shelled animals became trapped when the sand was soft and loose. Time passed. The sand hardened into rock. During this time, the soft parts of the animals vanished. But prints of their hard parts remained. Those prints are fossils.

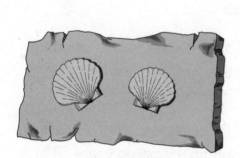 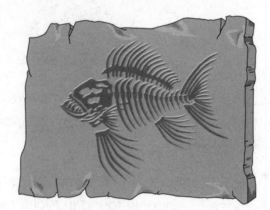

Some whole animals or plants are preserved in other ways. The fossil insect in the drawing was caught in sticky tree sap. The tree sap hardened, trapping the whole insect. Whole mammoths, which look like hairy elephants, have been found trapped in ice.

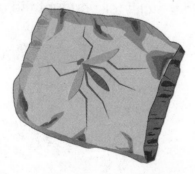

Now you know how some fossils form. What can they tell you about the past?

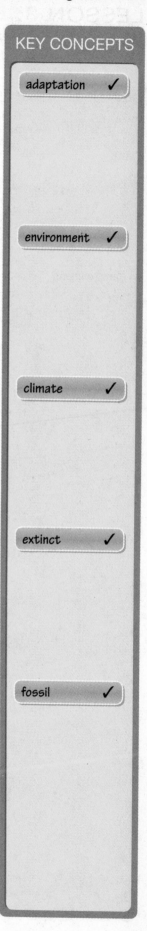

KEY CONCEPTS

adaptation ✓

environment ✓

climate ✓

extinct ✓

fossil ✓

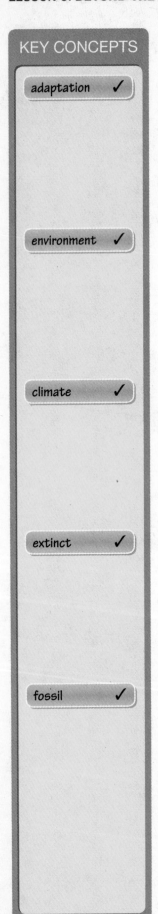

You're back in the present. Imagine that you are looking at the rocks that are on the beach now. What you see is shown in the drawing below. What can the fossils tell you?

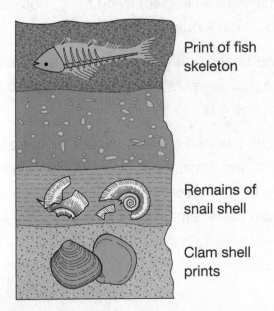

Print of fish skeleton

Remains of snail shell

Clam shell prints

Older fossils are in the lower layers of rock. Newer fossils are in the higher layers. Scientists can compare the fossils to see how living things changed over time.

Fossils also show that some forms of life became extinct. Fossils of dinosaurs are only found in rocks older than 65 million years. That means that dinosaurs became extinct about 65 million years ago. The environment changed then. Dinosaurs were not adapted to the new environment.

Fossils can also show that Earth has changed over time. The fish and shell fossils in the cliff tell you that the cliff was once under water.

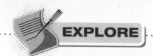

This drawing shows some rocks and fossils. Use the drawing to answer the questions.

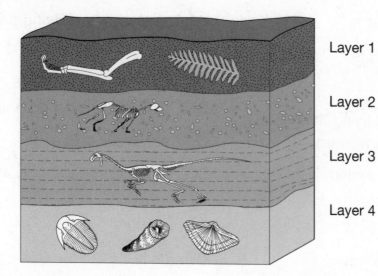

Layer 1

Layer 2

Layer 3

Layer 4

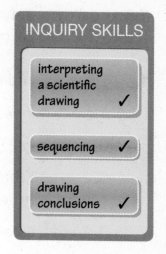

**INQUIRY SKILLS**

interpreting a scientific drawing ✓

sequencing ✓

drawing conclusions ✓

1. Which fossils are oldest?

_____

_____

2. Which fossils are youngest?

_____

_____

3. Which rock layer was once under water?

_____

_____

# PUTTING IT ALL TOGETHER

You are now ready to show you understand the key concepts covered in this topic. Read each question. Circle the letter of the best answer.

1. What is an adaptation?

   A. evidence of past life

   B. climate

   C. a trait that help a living thing to survive in its environment

   D. an animal that is extinct

2. Which of these adaptations protects a turtle?

   A. wings

   B. hard shell

   C. beak

   D. gills

3. Which is an adaptation of a sea bird?

   A. feathers that soak up water

   B. waterproof feathers

   C. no feathers

   D. feet without webs between the toes

4. What are some nonliving parts of a beach environment?

   A. air, water, and fish

   B. fish, crabs, and dolphins

   C. air, water, and sand

   D. birds, dune grasses, and air

5. Climate is

   A. the usual weather in a place.

   B. the unusual weather in a place.

   C. what a place looks like.

   D. a storm.

6. A living thing that is extinct is

   A. never gone from Earth.

   B. gone from Earth for a while.

   C. gone from Earth forever.

   D. alive.

**Use the drawings below to answer questions 7–10.**

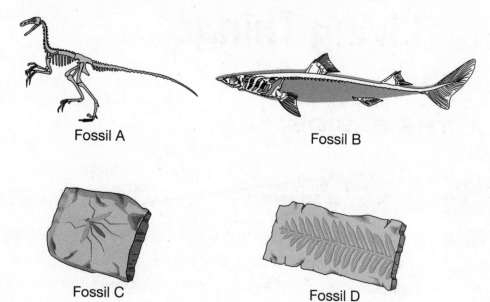

Fossil A

Fossil B

Fossil C

Fossil D

**7.** Which fossil is from an animal that walked on land?

    **A.** Fossil A

    **B.** Fossil B

    **C.** Fossil C

    **D.** Fossil D

**8.** Which fossil probably formed in water?

    **A.** Fossil A

    **B.** Fossil B

    **C.** Fossil C

    **D.** Fossil D

**9.** Which fossil is from an animal that could fly?

    **A.** Fossil A

    **B.** Fossil B

    **C.** Fossil C

    **D.** Fossil D

**10.** What made Fossil D?

    **A.** a land animal

    **B.** a plant

    **C.** a sea animal

    **D.** a person

# Understanding Living Things

## LESSON 1: **THE BASICS**

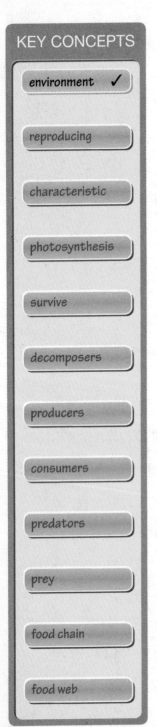

KEY CONCEPTS

environment ✓

reproducing

characteristic

photosynthesis

survive

decomposers

producers

consumers

predators

prey

food chain

food web

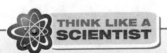

**THINK LIKE A SCIENTIST**

It is a hot summer day. You are visiting a park. Look around. What do you observe? The park is high above a wide river. Steep, rocky cliffs rise up from the river. Green grass covers the brown soil under your feet. A breeze moves the air through your hair. The sun shining on your skin is warm. You spy a hawk gliding through the air. A garter snake sliding under a bush startles you. You notice a cricket eating on a blade of grass. You almost trip on an old log covered with mushrooms. Everything you have just observed is part of the environment of the park. An **environment** includes all the living and nonliving things in a place.

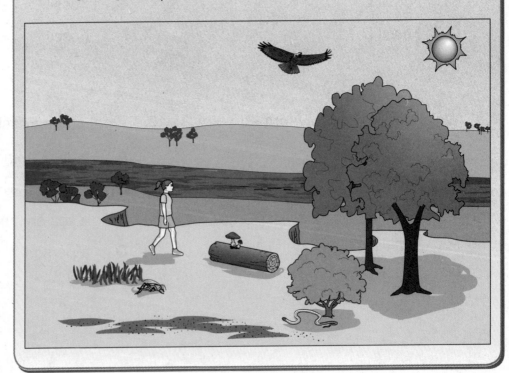

# What's Alive, What's Not

Sometimes it is easy to tell a living thing from a thing that is not alive. You are sure to know that a hawk, garter snake, and cricket are living things. They eat and they make little copies of themselves. The copies are young hawks, young garter snakes, and young crickets. Eating and reproducing are two of the things that living things do. **Reproducing** is to make more of one's own kind. All living things eat and reproduce. You know that a rock, a river, air, and sunshine are not living things. They do not eat anything. And they do not make little copies of themselves.

Is a mushroom alive? Is a blade of grass alive? You might not think so. You have never seen a mushroom or blade of grass eating. And you have never seen a mushroom or blade of grass make little mushrooms or little blades of grass.

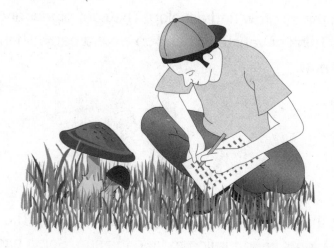

Look at the list on the next page. It shows the characteristics of living things. A **characteristic** may be something that an object does or it may be one of its parts. The list will help you decide whether a mushroom, blade of grass, or any other object is alive.

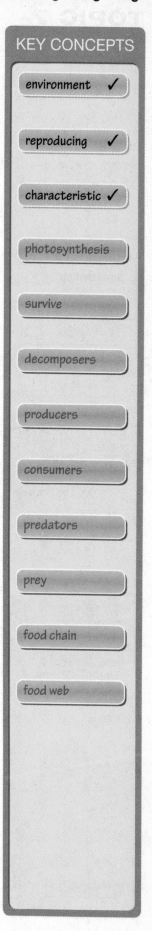

KEY CONCEPTS

environment ✓

reproducing ✓

characteristic ✓

photosynthesis

survive

decomposers

producers

consumers

predators

prey

food chain

food web

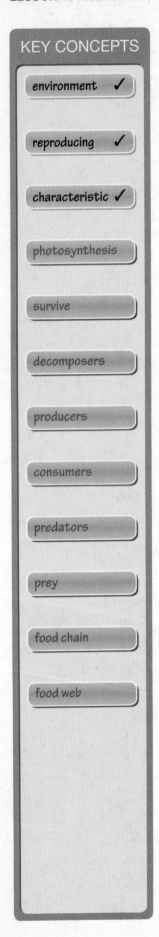

# Characteristics of Living Things

- All living things are made of cells. Cells are tiny parts of living things. You have to use a microscope to see most cells.

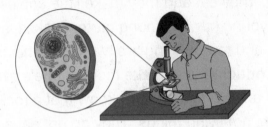

- All living things take in or make their own food. Animals eat food. Plants make their own food. Mushrooms take in dead parts of plants and animals.

- All living things get rid of wastes. Animals get rid of solid wastes and liquid wastes. Plants get rid of wastes that are gases.

- All living things grow and develop. They get bigger and they change. Think of yourself when you were a baby. Then think of yourself now.

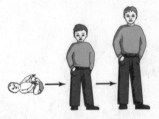

- All living things respond to changes around them. The stems of some plants keep turning to face the sun. Some birds fly to where it is warm when cold winter days come.

- All living things reproduce. They make more living things like themselves. Think of a nest of young hawks. Think of apple trees growing from apple seeds.

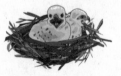

- Most living things, or their parts, move. Think of a hawk flying. Leaves have little holes that open and close to let air and water in and out.

102

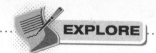

EXPLORE

The picture below shows the park you have been reading about. Objects in the picture are numbered. Make checkmarks in the boxes below that describe what the object does. Finally, write "living" or "nonliving" in the boxes in the column headed "Conclusion."

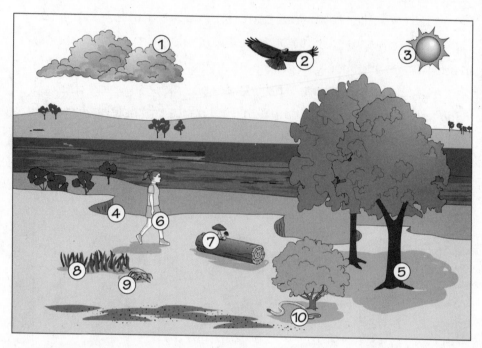
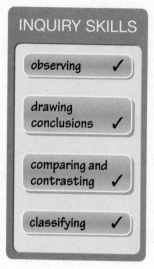

| Object | Has Cells | Takes in or Makes Own Food | Gets Rid of Wastes | Grows and Develops | Responds to Changes in the Environment | Reproduces | Moves or Parts Move | Conclusion |
|---|---|---|---|---|---|---|---|---|
| 1. | | | | | | | ✓ | nonliving |
| 2. | ✓ | ✓ | ✓ | ✓ | ✓ | ✓ | ✓ | living |
| 3. | | | | | | | | |
| 4. | | | | | | | | |
| 5. | | | | | | | | |
| 6. | | | | | | | | |
| 7. | | | | | | | | |
| 8. | | | | | | | | |
| 9. | | | | | | | | |
| 10. | | | | | | | | |

# LESSON 2: **BUILDING ON THE BASICS**

## KEY CONCEPTS

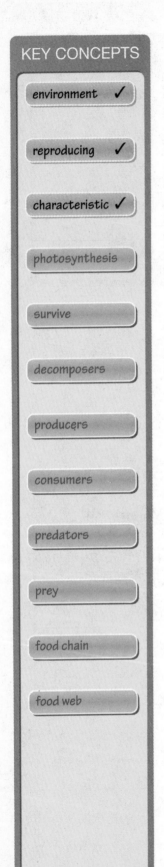

environment ✓

reproducing ✓

characteristic ✓

photosynthesis

survive

decomposers

producers

consumers

predators

prey

food chain

food web

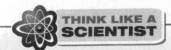
**THINK LIKE A SCIENTIST**

It is very warm in the park. You have just climbed a steep hill. You are out of breath. So you take a deep breath of air. You are also thirsty. So you drink water from your canteen. You are a little hungry, too. So you munch on a carrot you have taken along in your backpack. In one way or another, you have just interacted with the nonliving parts of the environment. And you are not alone in doing that. All living things interact with the nonliving parts of their environment. Hawks do. So do snakes and crickets. So do grasses, all other plants, and even mushrooms. Nonliving parts of the environment make life possible on Earth. But how do they do this?

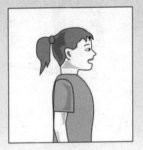 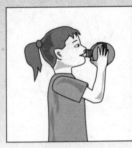 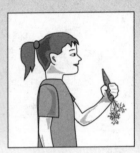

## Living Things Need Air

You cannot see the air in the park. But it holds three things that living things need. These things are oxygen, carbon dioxide, and water vapor. Each of these is a colorless gas. That is why you cannot see them.

You and all animals need oxygen. You take in oxygen with each breath of air. Your blood takes the oxygen to your cells. Your cells use the oxygen to change food into energy. Your body uses the energy to move. Your body also uses the energy for all its other activities.

Plants need carbon dioxide to make their food. You will learn more about this on page 106.

The water vapor in air can change into droplets of liquid water. The droplets can form clouds. Rain, snow, sleet, and hail can fall from the clouds. Living things need this water to stay alive.

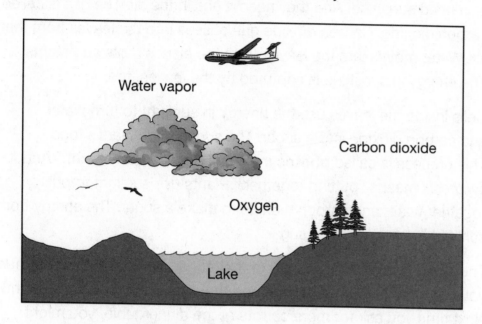

## Living Things Need Water

The cells of all living things make chemicals. You and all living things need these chemicals to stay alive. One chemical helps you grow. Another helps you see. Another chemical helps send messages along your nerves. Your body needs chemicals to move and to digest food. Your body makes thousands of chemicals. It needs water to make these chemicals. So you and all other living things must take in water.

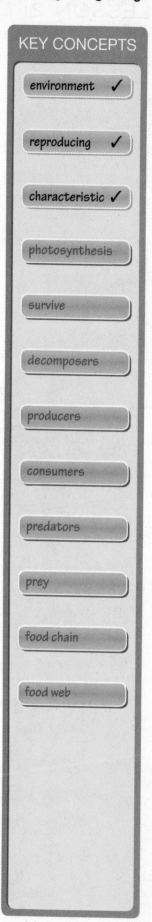

KEY CONCEPTS

environment ✓

reproducing ✓

characteristic ✓

photosynthesis

survive

decomposers

producers

consumers

predators

prey

food chain

food web

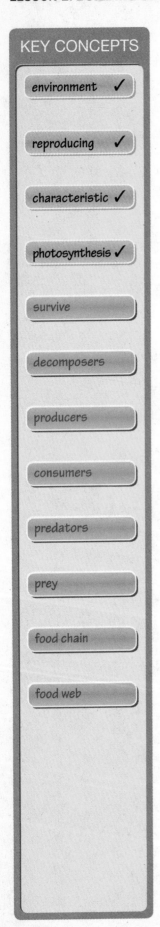

# Plants Need Soil and Sunshine

Plants need water to make their own food. But to do this job, they also need sunshine. And they need a gas in the air. The gas is called carbon dioxide. Carbon dioxide gas passes into the leaves from the air. Water moves into the leaves from the plant's roots and stems. The energy in sunshine is captured by the leaves, too.

Cells inside the leaves use the energy in sunlight to turn water and carbon dioxide into a sugar. The sugar is the plant's food. This process is called **photosynthesis**. *Photo* means "light." And *synthesis* means "putting together." Plants use sunlight to put together water and carbon dioxide to make a sugar. The energy from sunlight is trapped in the sugar.

The carrot you ate holds some of that sugar. So what happens when you eat a carrot? You take in a food that holds energy from sunlight. Next time you ask for more carrots at the dinner table, you might say, "Pass me some sunshine."

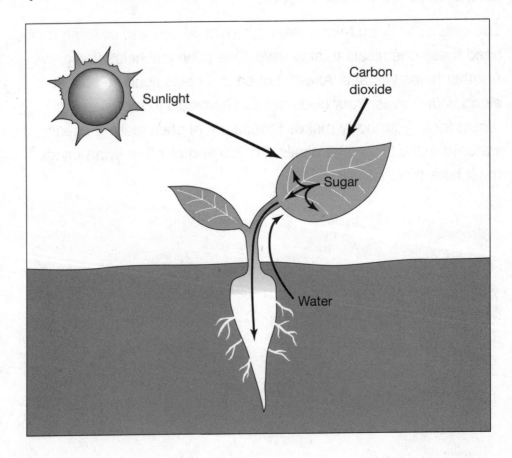

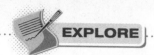

Plants stay alive by using nonliving things in their environment. The drawing below shows a plant and its parts. The arrows show the paths nonliving things take into the plant. Next to each arrow, write the name of the thing that is going into that part of the plant. On the lines below the picture, tell how the plant uses nonliving things to make its food.

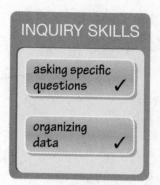

INQUIRY SKILLS

asking specific questions ✓

organizing data ✓

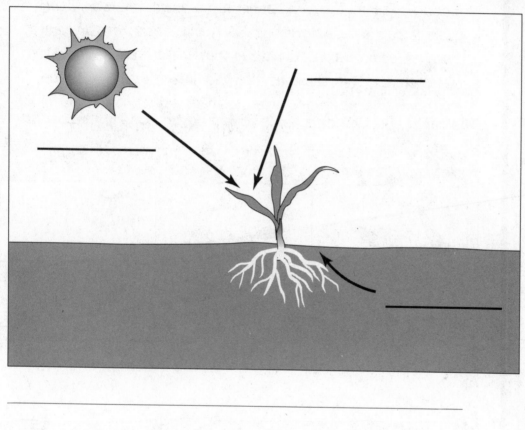

_____

_____

_____

# LESSON 3: **BEYOND THE BASICS**

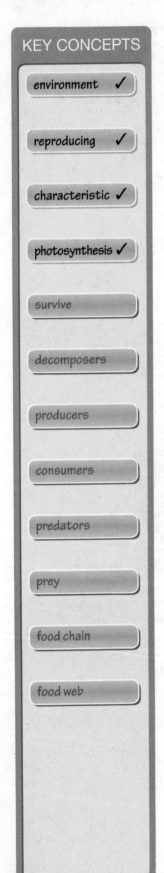
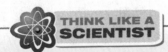

**THINK LIKE A SCIENTIST**

Watch that hawk. It seems to be gliding lazily in the air. But it is really on the hunt. It is looking for a meal on the ground. The garter snake has come out from under the bush. It is on the hunt, too. It is headed for the cricket nibbling on a blade of grass. The grass is the cricket's food. The mushrooms on the rotting log are a kind of clean-up team. They are cleaning up dead bits of wood. Other mushrooms are cleaning up the dead parts of crickets and leaves. The mushrooms are breaking down the dead materials. When the mushrooms do this, they put food back into the soil. The grass uses some of that food to grow. All these activities provide food and energy for the park's living things. These activities form patterns. What kinds of patterns? That is for you to discover.

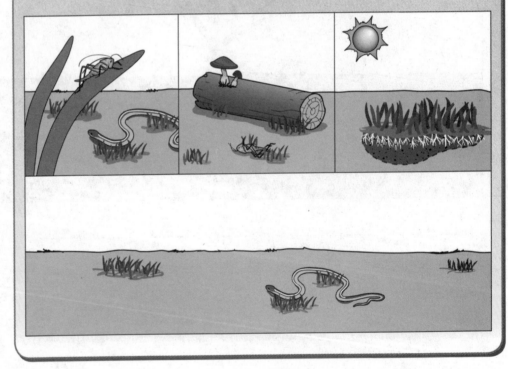

# The Roles of Living Things

Living things in an environment need other living things to **survive**. To survive means to stay alive. All living things need food. One way scientists group living things is by how they get food.

- **Decomposers** get food by breaking down the dead parts of plants and animals. They also put foods back into the soil that plants need. Mushrooms are decomposers.

- **Producers** make their own food. Plants are producers.

- **Consumers** eat plants. They also eat animals that eat plants. Crickets, garter snakes, and hawks are consumers.

- **Predators** are consumers that eat other animals. Hawks and snakes are predators.

- **Prey** are consumers that predators eat. A cricket is the prey of a garter snake. And a garter snake is the prey of a hawk.

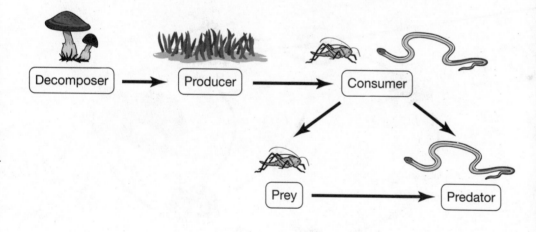

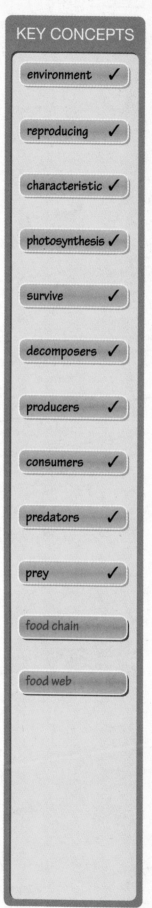

KEY CONCEPTS

environment ✓

reproducing ✓

characteristic ✓

photosynthesis ✓

survive ✓

decomposers ✓

producers ✓

consumers ✓

predators ✓

prey ✓

food chain

food web

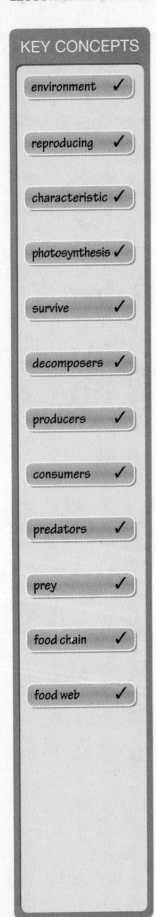

KEY CONCEPTS

environment ✓

reproducing ✓

characteristic ✓

photosynthesis ✓

survive ✓

decomposers ✓

producers ✓

consumers ✓

predators ✓

prey ✓

food chain ✓

food web ✓

## Food Chains

The living things you have seen in the park form a food chain. A **food chain** shows how food passes from one living thing to another in an environment. Look at the picture. It shows the food chain you observed in the park. Each living thing in the food chain provides food for the next living thing in the chain.

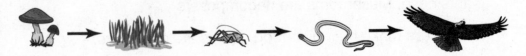

## Food Webs

There are many food chains in an environment. Some food chains are connected to each other. A set of connected food chains makes a **food web**. A food web shows the different ways food is passed among living things in an environment.

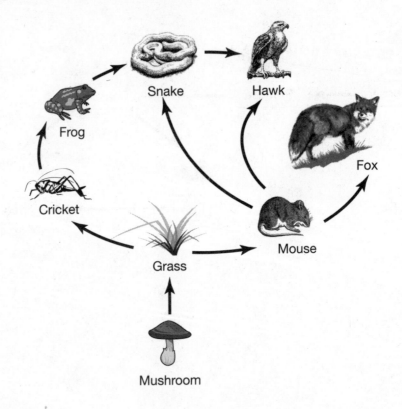

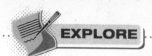

Study the food web on the opposite page. The living things in the food web are listed in the left-most column in the chart below. Place a check mark in the boxes that identify the role of each living thing in the food web. An animal can be both prey and predator.

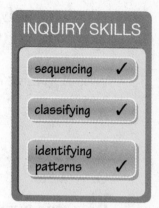

| Living Thing | Decomposer | Producer | Consumer | Predator | Prey |
|---|---|---|---|---|---|
| Mushroom | | | | | |
| Grass | | | | | |
| Cricket | | | | | |
| Frog | | | | | |
| Snake | | | | | |
| Hawk | | | | | |
| Mouse | | | | | |
| Fox | | | | | |

# PUTTING IT ALL TOGETHER

**You are now ready to show you understand the key concepts covered in this topic. Read each question. Circle the letter of the best answer.**

1. Which is alive?

   A. soil

   B. air

   C. water

   D. rose bush

2. Which sentence is correct?

   A. Some living things reproduce.

   B. All living things reproduce.

   C. No living things reproduce.

   D. A few living things reproduce.

3. What do plants use to get energy to make food?

   A. water

   B. air

   C. sunshine

   D. soil

4. What is photosynthesis?

   A. a picture

   B. the way plants make food

   C. sunlight

   D. the way plants use food

5. Which is a consumer?

   A. cow

   B. peach tree

   C. mushroom

   D. grass

6.  Which set of pictures shows a food chain in the right order?

A.
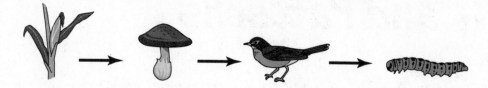

B.
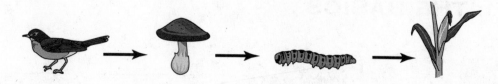

C.
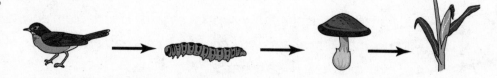

D.
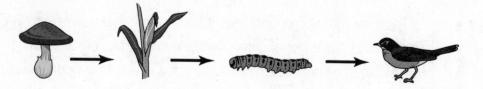

7.  Which is a producer?

A.  cricket

B.  mushroom

C.  hawk

D.  rose bush

8.  All living things

A.  make their own food.

B.  eat other living things.

C.  need water.

D.  get food from soil.

# Earth's Cycles and Patterns

## LESSON 1: **THE BASICS**

**KEY CONCEPTS**

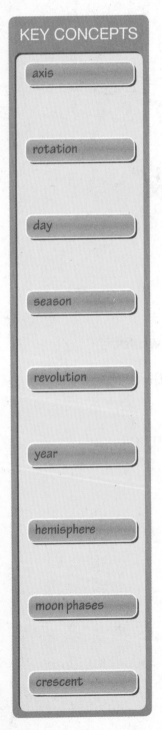

axis

rotation

day

season

revolution

year

hemisphere

moon phases

crescent

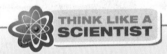
**THINK LIKE A SCIENTIST**

It's early evening. You look out your window. The sun is setting. In the distance, where the sky meets the ground, the clouds turn pink. Gradually, the pink color fades to gray. At last the sun has set. Stars pop out of the darkening sky.

You have just watched day turn into night. Hours from now, night will turn into day again. You know that this pattern repeats over and over. But how does it happen?

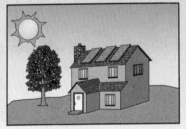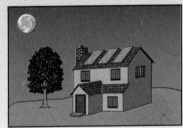

## Day and Night

To you it seems as though Earth is standing still. But Earth is moving all the time. To you it seems as if objects in the sky are moving. After all, you see the sun come up in the east every morning. During the day, it crosses the sky. And it sets in the west every evening. The stars also move across the sky from east to west. But your eyes are fooling you. Here is what is really happening.

To see what is really happening, you might have to get away from Earth. Think of what it would be like to be in outer space! You see planet Earth in front of you. It looks like a huge blue and white ball. You notice right away that Earth is spinning. It spins around its axis. Earth's **axis** is an imaginary line that Earth spins around. The axis is like a rod that goes through Earth from its North Pole to its South Pole. Earth spins like a top.

The drawing below shows Earth's axis. You can see that the axis does not go straight up and down. Instead, Earth is tilted on its axis.

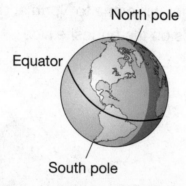

North pole

Equator

South pole

The place where the axis meets Earth's surface is called a *pole*. Earth has a North Pole and a South Pole.

Earth's spinning motion is called **rotation**. The arrow in the drawing below shows the direction of Earth's rotation. Earth rotates from west to east.

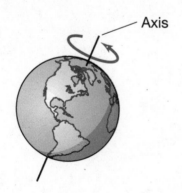

Axis

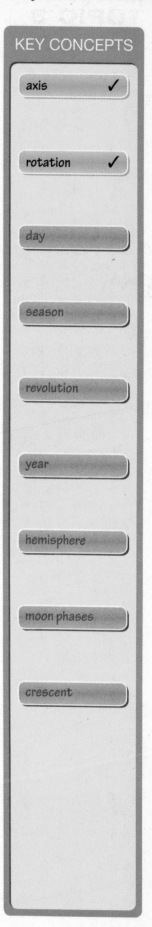

KEY CONCEPTS

axis ✓

rotation ✓

day

season

revolution

year

hemisphere

moon phases

crescent

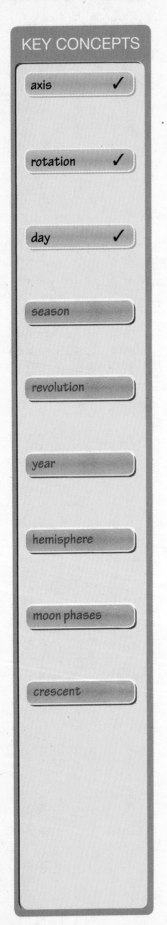

KEY CONCEPTS

axis ✓

rotation ✓

day ✓

season

revolution

year

hemisphere

moon phases

crescent

It takes Earth one day, or 24 hours, to make one rotation. A **day** is one rotation of Earth.

As Earth rotates, half of its surface faces the sun. The other half faces away from the sun. The half facing the sun is lit up. It's daytime on this half of Earth. The half that faces away from the sun is dark. It's nighttime on that side. As Earth continues to rotate, daytime and nighttime come to different parts of Earth.

Look at the drawing. It shows North America and South America in daylight. Places on the opposite side of the world are in darkness. As the world turns, night will come to North and South America. And day will come to places on the opposite side.

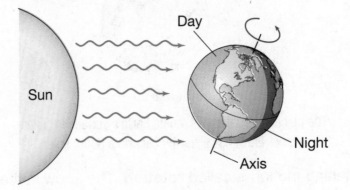

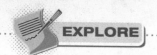 **EXPLORE**

Here's a way to explore Earth's daylight and nighttime cycle. Find a small flashlight to be your model sun. Find a ball to be your model Earth. The ball should be about the size of a softball.

Have a friend or relative hold the flashlight "sun" in the middle of a darkened room. Have the person turn on the flashlight. Hold "Earth" about one foot in front of the shining "sun." Slowly spin "Earth" to model rotation.

See how rotation causes day and night. Draw and label your model in the space below. Then write two or three sentences to explain what causes day and night.

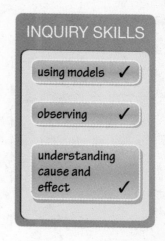

INQUIRY SKILLS

using models ✓

observing ✓

understanding cause and effect ✓

# LESSON 2: BUILDING ON THE BASICS

## KEY CONCEPTS

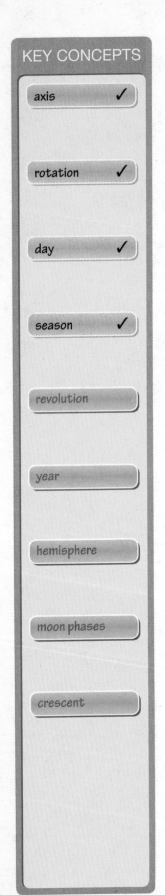

- axis ✓
- rotation ✓
- day ✓
- season ✓
- revolution
- year
- hemisphere
- moon phases
- crescent

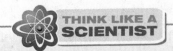

**THINK LIKE A SCIENTIST**

Back on Earth again, you find yourself sitting beside your window. Outside, leaves are falling from the trees. In a few months, snow will cover the grass. In a few more months, warmer weather will come. Flowers will bud. Still later, the warmest days of the year will come. Then the cycle will repeat. You will have seen Earth's four seasons come and go.

A **season** is a part of the year with a certain kind of weather. Fall, winter, spring, and summer are seasons. Like day and night, seasons are part of a cycle. You already know that Earth's rotation causes day and night. You ask yourself, "What causes Earth's seasons?"

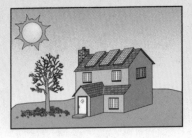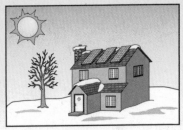

## Seasons

To see how seasons are caused, you need to get away from Earth again. If you go far enough, you can see both the sun and Earth. You can see that Earth's tilt makes one of its poles lean toward the sun. You can also see that Earth is not just spinning. It is moving around the sun!

Earth's movement around the sun is called **revolution**. It takes Earth about 365 days to make one revolution around the sun. One revolution around the sun equals one **year**. So a year is about 365 days long.

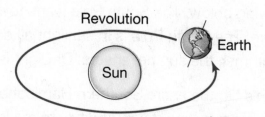

As you watch Earth revolve, you see the seasons changing in its top and bottom halves. These halves are called **hemispheres**. The Northern Hemisphere is the half that is in the north. The Southern Hemisphere is the half that is in the south. The United States is in the Northern Hemisphere.

Look at Earth at point A. At this point, the Northern Hemisphere tilts away from the sun. That part of Earth is having winter. At the same time, the Southern Hemisphere tilts toward the sun. That part of Earth is having summer.

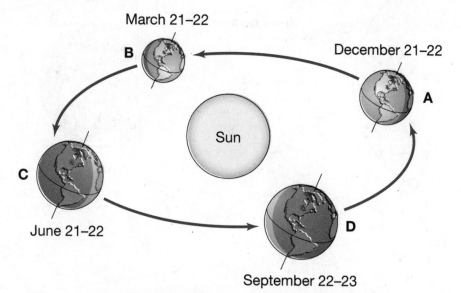

At point C, the Northern Hemisphere is having summer.
The Southern Hemisphere is having winter.
At point D, the Northern Hemisphere is having autumn.
The Southern Hemisphere is having spring.
The seasons are always opposite in opposite hemispheres.

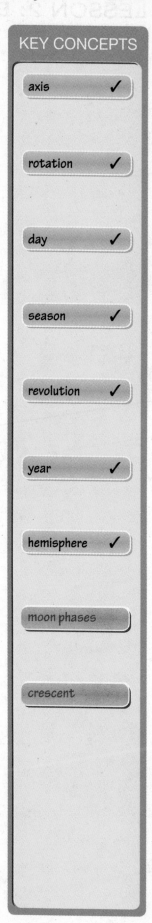

KEY CONCEPTS

axis ✓

rotation ✓

day ✓

season ✓

revolution ✓

year ✓

hemisphere ✓

moon phases

crescent

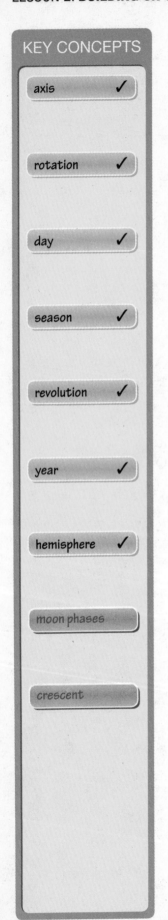

axis ✓

rotation ✓

day ✓

season ✓

revolution ✓

year ✓

hemisphere ✓

moon phases

crescent

What do you suppose people mean when they say that summer days are long? After all, a day in summer lasts 24 hours. A day in winter lasts 24 hours, too. When they say a day is long, they are really talking about daylight being long.

Look at the drawing below. The South Pole leans toward the sun. It is summer there. The South Pole is in sunlight all day long. At the South Pole in summer, the sun never sets. Daylight is very long.

Because of Earth's tilt, the entire Southern Hemisphere is in daylight for more than 12 hours a day. Hours of daylight are long. The sun sets late and rises early.

Now look at the North Pole. The North Pole leans away from the sun. It is winter there. The North Pole is in darkness all day long. At the North Pole in winter, the sun never rises. Night is very long.

Because of Earth's tilt, the entire Northern Hemisphere is in darkness for more than 12 hours a day. Hours of daylight are short. The sun sets early and rises late.

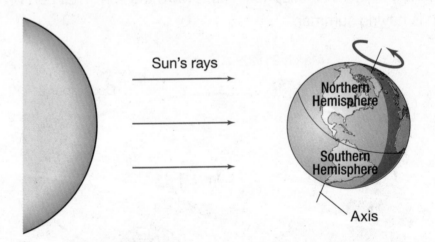

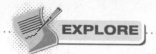 **EXPLORE**

Use a small flashlight to represent the sun. Use a globe to represent Earth. Notice that the globe is tilted on its axis.

Find the United States. Have someone hold the "sun" in the middle of a darkened room. Hold the globe about one foot in front of the shining "sun."

Slowly move the globe around the "sun" to model revolution. **NOTE: Make sure the globe always tilts in the same direction as you move it around the "sun."** For example, the globe could always be tilted towards the door to the room.

In the space below, draw and label each position of the globe that causes a different season in the United States. Label the seasons. Then write two or three sentences to explain what causes seasons. Remember: spring follows winter, summer follows spring, fall follows summer, and winter follows fall.

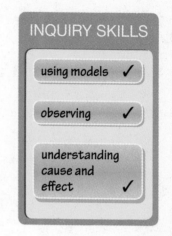

INQUIRY SKILLS

using models ✓

observing ✓

understanding cause and effect ✓

# LESSON 3: **BEYOND THE BASICS**

## KEY CONCEPTS

axis ✓

rotation ✓

day ✓

season ✓

revolution ✓

year ✓

hemisphere ✓

moon phases

crescent

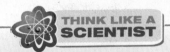
**THINK LIKE A SCIENTIST**

You are at your bedroom window. It is night. You look outside and observe the moon. It is shaped like a complete circle. That's odd, you think. A few nights ago it was less than a complete circle. And last week, it looked like a half circle. The week before that you could not see it at all. You think, "The moon seems to change its shape as time passes." You guess that the moon isn't really changing shape. It only looks as if it is doing that. You ask yourself, "What makes the moon look as if it's changing shape?"

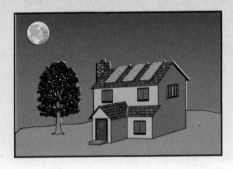

## Moon Phases

To answer your question, you have to discover how the moon moves. To do that, you have to go back into space. There you see Earth revolving around the sun. At the same time, you see the moon revolving around Earth. Earth and the moon move together around the sun.

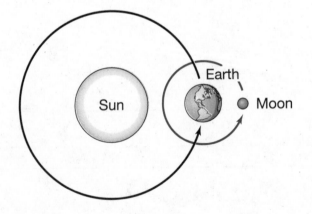

122

Now move to a point in space above both the moon and Earth. Looking down, you would see something like the drawing below. No matter where the moon is as it travels around Earth, half of it is always in sunlight. All that changes is which part.

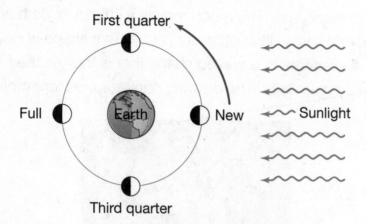

But seen from Earth, the moon seems to change shape as it goes around Earth. These changes are called **moon phases**. The drawing below shows what the moon looks like from Earth at four points in its revolution.

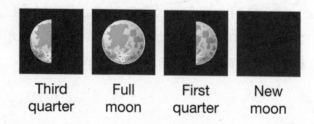

| Third quarter | Full moon | First quarter | New moon |

What has changed? The portion of the moon that reflects sunlight to Earth.

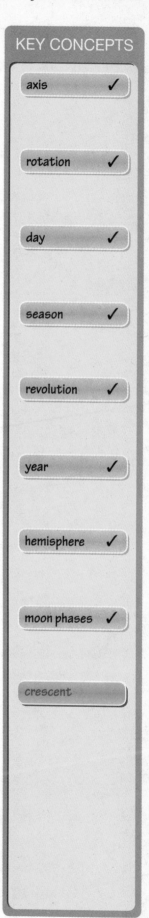

KEY CONCEPTS

axis ✓

rotation ✓

day ✓

season ✓

revolution ✓

year ✓

hemisphere ✓

moon phases ✓

crescent

123

**KEY CONCEPTS**

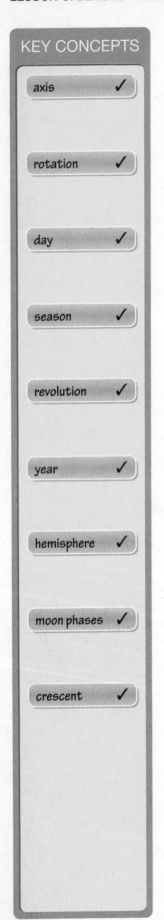

axis ✓

rotation ✓

day ✓

season ✓

revolution ✓

year ✓

hemisphere ✓

moon phases ✓

crescent ✓

The cycle of moon phases starts with the new moon. Look at the drawings on the previous page. The moon is between Earth and the sun at that point. The moon's sunlit half is facing away from us. We cannot see the moon. Only its dark side is facing us.

A couple of days pass. The moon moves a little in its path around Earth. You can see a sliver of its sunlit half. This shape is called a crescent. A **crescent** is a curved shape that is thick in the middle and pointed on its ends. The drawing shows a crescent moon.

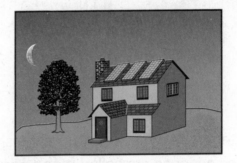

In about a week you can see more of the sunlit half of the moon. The moon is in its first-quarter phase. It looks like a half-moon!

Another week passes. The moon is full. You can see all of its sunlit half. It takes about one month for the moon to go through all its phases. Then the cycle starts over.

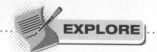 EXPLORE

You can model the phases of the moon. Use a small flashlight to model the sun. Use a medium-size ball to model Earth. Use a small ball to model the moon.

Have someone hold the "sun" on one side of a darkened room. Hold "Earth" about two feet in front of the shining sun. Put the "moon" between "Earth" and the "sun." Have a fourth person, the "observer," stand behind "Earth" opposite the "moon." This person will observe that none of the lit side of the "moon" can be seen from "Earth."

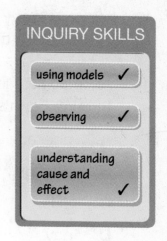

INQUIRY SKILLS

using models ✓

observing ✓

understanding cause and effect ✓

Move the "moon" to its first-quarter position. The observer should face the "moon" from the opposite side of "Earth." How much of the "moon" is visible at this position? Repeat this two more times, once at full moon position and once at third-quarter position. Always have the observer move to the side of "Earth" opposite the "moon."

Draw and label each moon phase in your model in the space below. Then write two or three sentences to explain what causes moon phases.

# PUTTING IT ALL TOGETHER

**You are now ready to show you understand the key concepts covered in this topic. Read each question. Circle the letter of the best answer.**

1.  An imaginary line that runs through Earth's poles is called a(n)

    A.  phase.

    B.  rotation.

    C.  axis.

    D.  day.

2.  Spinning around an axis is called

    A.  revolution.

    B.  rotation.

    C.  month.

    D.  year.

3.  What causes day and night?

    A.  Earth's rotation

    B.  Earth's revolution

    C.  first-quarter moon

    D.  third-quarter moon

4.  A time of year with certain weather is a

    A.  hemisphere.

    B.  revolution.

    C.  phase.

    D.  season.

5.  What causes seasons?

    A.  Earth's rotation

    B.  Earth's revolution

    C.  Earth's rotation and its tilt

    D.  Earth's revolution and its tilt

6.  When it is spring in the Northern Hemisphere, what season is it in the Southern Hemisphere?

    A.  spring

    B.  summer

    C.  fall

    D.  winter

7. Days in the Northern Hemisphere have more hours of daylight during

   A. July.

   B. January.

   C. April.

   D. October.

8. How much of the moon's surface is always in sunlight?

   A. one-quarter

   B. one-half

   C. three-quarters

   D. all

9. The changes in the shape of Earth's moon as seen from Earth are

   A. revolutions.

   B. rotations.

   C. phases.

   D. seasons.

10. You cannot see the moon in the sky during the

    A. new moon.

    B. first-quarter moon.

    C. full moon.

    D. third-quarter moon.

# TOPIC 9   Weather

## LESSON 1: **THE BASICS**

### KEY CONCEPTS

weather ✓

precipitation

water cycle

evaporation

condensation

thermometer

anemometer

air pressure

barometer

warm front

cold front

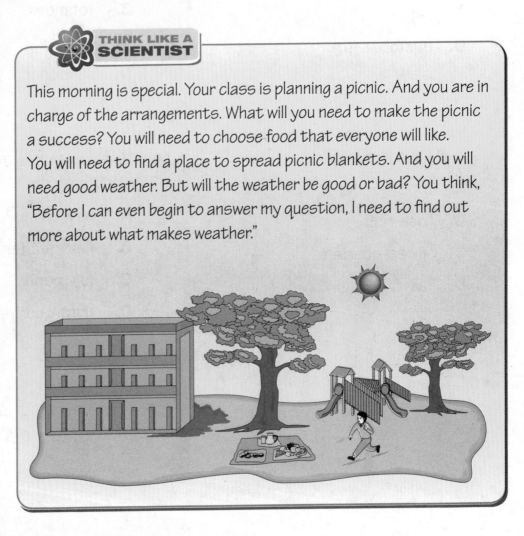

**THINK LIKE A SCIENTIST**

This morning is special. Your class is planning a picnic. And you are in charge of the arrangements. What will you need to make the picnic a success? You will need to choose food that everyone will like. You will need to find a place to spread picnic blankets. And you will need good weather. But will the weather be good or bad? You think, "Before I can even begin to answer my question, I need to find out more about what makes weather."

## Water in the Air

**Weather** is what the air is like around you. The air can be cool or warm. It can be clear or full of clouds. It can be windy or quiet. It can be dry or wet. Water can even fall from it. And that wouldn't be good for your picnic.

On a clear morning, you might think that there was no water in the air. But there is always water in the air. How does it get there? And what can happen to it? The answers to these questions may help you decide whether today is a good day for your picnic.

128

There is always some water in the air. If there is lots of it up there, it might come down as rain, snow, sleet, or hail. Rain, snow, sleet, and hail are called precipitation. **Precipitation** is water that falls from the sky.

Snow and hail are solid precipitation. They are forms of ice. Rain is liquid precipitation. And sleet is a combination of liquid and solid precipitation.

What turns water into different kinds of precipitation? Water in the air can change form. It can be a liquid if the air is warm. It can freeze solid if the air is cold. It can also be a gas that you cannot see. That gas is called water vapor.

Clouds are made of water vapor. There is also water vapor in a sky without clouds. On a clear day, the bits of water are too far apart to see.

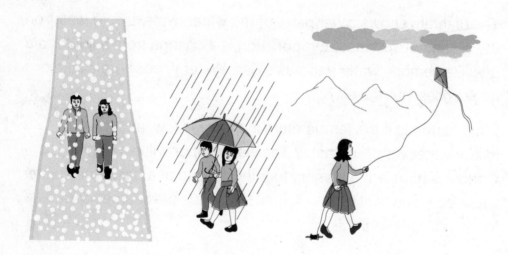

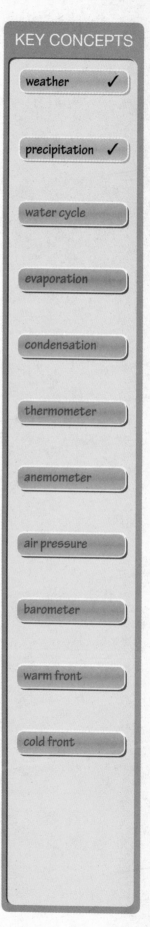

KEY CONCEPTS

weather ✓

precipitation ✓

water cycle

evaporation

condensation

thermometer

anemometer

air pressure

barometer

warm front

cold front

Precipitation is part of the water cycle. The **water cycle** moves water from the land and sea into the air and back again. Look at the diagram. Find precipitation.

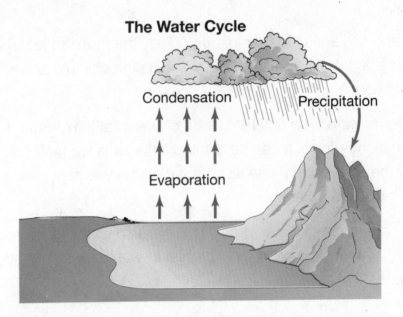

**The Water Cycle**

Condensation

Precipitation

Evaporation

The diagram shows other parts of the water cycle. Liquid water on the ground evaporates. **Evaporation** is a change from a liquid to a gas. Remember, water vapor is a gas. Water vapor from a lake or ocean rises into the air.

What happens if the temperature in the air is low, and there is lots of water vapor up there? The water vapor will condense. **Condensation** is the coming together of bits of a gas. When water vapor condenses, it forms clouds. If it condenses some more, it forms precipitation.

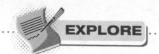 **EXPLORE**

In the chart below, make a record of the weather during the next three days. Write down what you observe in the morning, and again in the afternoon. Here are some questions you can answer:

- Is the sky clear or cloudy? What do the clouds look like?

- How does the air feel? Is it warm or cool? Is it damp or dry?

- Is it windy or still? Are the winds strong or light?

- Is there precipitation? What kind of precipitation is it? How much precipitation is there?

At the end of the third day, look back at your records for all three days. Has the weather changed? If it has, how has it changed? Write answers to these two questions on the lines below the chart.

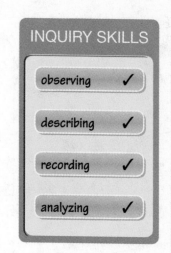

INQUIRY SKILLS

| observing | ✓ |
| describing | ✓ |
| recording | ✓ |
| analyzing | ✓ |

| WEATHER RECORD | |
|---|---|
| **Morning** | **Afternoon** |
| Day 1 | |
| Day 2 | |
| Day 3 | |

_____

_____

_____

_____

# LESSON 2: **BUILDING ON THE BASICS**

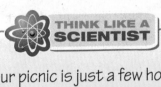

**THINK LIKE A SCIENTIST**

Your picnic is just a few hours away. You and your classmates are getting excited. You keep an eye on the sky as you think about your picnic. During each recess, you look at the sky and feel the air. Will it be too cold for your picnic? Will it be too warm? Will it be too windy? Will it rain?

You can see and feel the weather all around you. But you ask yourself, "Are there ways I can measure what I observe? And can these measurements help me predict the weather for the picnic?"

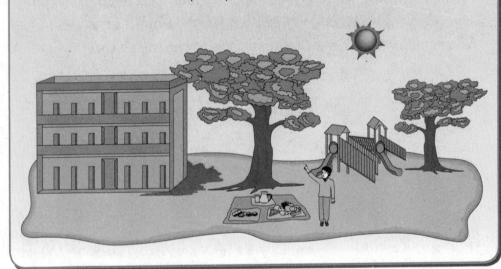

## How Weather Factors Are Measured

When you're having a picnic, you don't want the weather to be too hot or too cold. You can find out if it's hot or cold by measuring the temperature with a **thermometer**. Thermometers use two different temperature scales. These are called Celsius and Fahrenheit. Scientists use the Celsius scale. A television or radio weather person will most often use the Fahrenheit scale. The drawing shows the two temperature scales side by side.

A comfortable air temperature is about 22 degrees Celsius (22°C). That's the same as 72 degrees Fahrenheit (72°F). Water freezes at 0°C, or 32°F. It boils at 100°C, or 212°F.

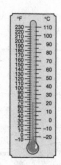

Where might a change in the weather be coming from? A wind vane can tell you. A wind vane shows which way the wind is blowing. And a change in the weather often comes on the wind.

A wind vane can turn freely in the wind. The part that turns is often shaped like an arrow. The arrow always points in the direction from which the wind is coming.

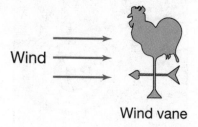

Wind

Wind vane

An **anemometer** shows how fast the wind is blowing. Instead of an arrow, it has cups on arms that reach out into the wind. As the wind blows, the cups spin around a rod. The faster the wind blows, the faster the cups spin. An instrument attached to the anemometer tells how fast the wind is blowing.

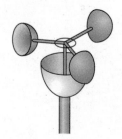

KEY CONCEPTS

weather ✓

precipitation ✓

water cycle ✓

evaporation ✓

condensation ✓

thermometer ✓

anemometer ✓

air pressure

barometer

warm front

cold front

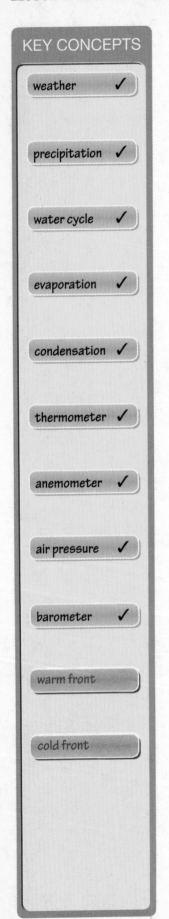

KEY CONCEPTS

- weather ✓
- precipitation ✓
- water cycle ✓
- evaporation ✓
- condensation ✓
- thermometer ✓
- anemometer ✓
- air pressure ✓
- barometer ✓
- warm front
- cold front

You can't feel it, but air has weight! It presses down against Earth's surface. This weight is called **air pressure**.

A **barometer** is a tool that measures air pressure. A change in air pressure often means a change in the weather.

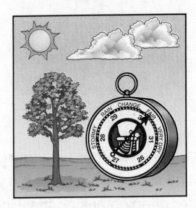

Rising pressure usually means you can expect fair weather.

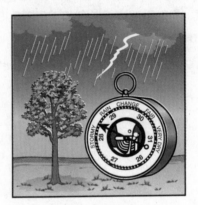

When the pressure drops, a storm may be coming your way.

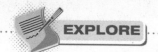 **EXPLORE**

Make a record of the weather during the next three days. This time, record the wind direction, wind speed, and air pressure. You can find this information in a TV weather report, in a newspaper, or on the Internet. Record the weather in the morning and the afternoon.

At the end of the third day, look back at your data. Has the weather changed? Did the data hint that it would change? Write your answers on the lines below the chart.

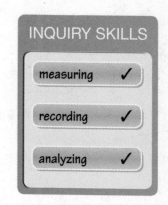

**INQUIRY SKILLS**

| measuring | ✓ |
| recording | ✓ |
| analyzing | ✓ |

| WEATHER RECORD | | |
|---|---|---|
| | **Morning** | **Afternoon** |
| Day 1 Wind direction | | |
| Wind speed | | |
| Air pressure | | |
| Weather | | |
| Day 2 Wind direction | | |
| Wind speed | | |
| Air pressure | | |
| Weather | | |
| Day 3 Wind direction | | |
| Wind speed | | |
| Air pressure | | |
| Weather | | |

_____

_____

_____

_____

_____

# LESSON 3: **BEYOND THE BASICS**

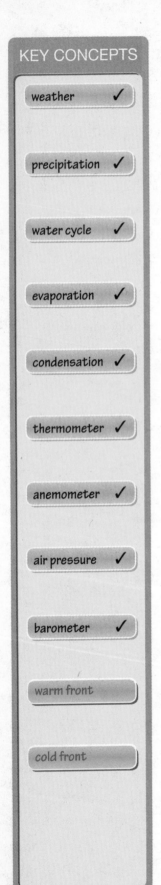

KEY CONCEPTS

weather ✓

precipitation ✓

water cycle ✓

evaporation ✓

condensation ✓

thermometer ✓

anemometer ✓

air pressure ✓

barometer ✓

warm front

cold front

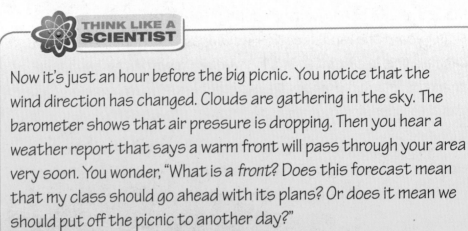

**THINK LIKE A SCIENTIST**

Now it's just an hour before the big picnic. You notice that the wind direction has changed. Clouds are gathering in the sky. The barometer shows that air pressure is dropping. Then you hear a weather report that says a warm front will pass through your area very soon. You wonder, "What is a *front*? Does this forecast mean that my class should go ahead with its plans? Or does it mean we should put off the picnic to another day?"

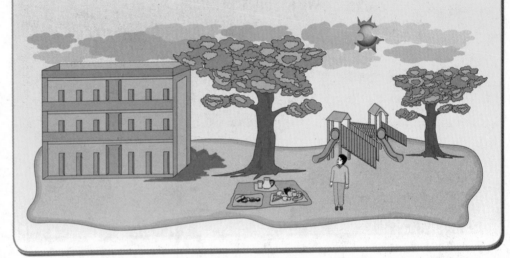

## Predicting Weather

Weather often changes where chunks of cool air meet chunks of warm air. These chunks of air are called air masses. A front is where air masses meet. Fronts often bring rain or snow. Wind speed and wind direction often change. The air may become warmer or cooler, and wetter or dryer.

A **warm front** often pushes clouds and rain ahead of it. Rainfall becomes heavier as the front moves closer. Sometimes a warm front brings fog. Sometimes it brings thunderstorms. Warmer air and clearing skies follow a warm front.

### Warm Front

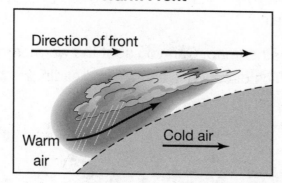

A **cold front** travels faster than a warm front. The weather changes more quickly. The precipitation that travels with the front is over sooner. Cooler air follows a cold front. In winter, the front can be followed by chilly temperatures.

### Cold Front

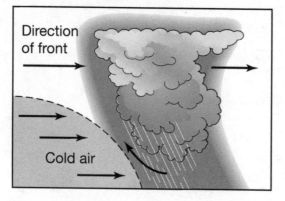

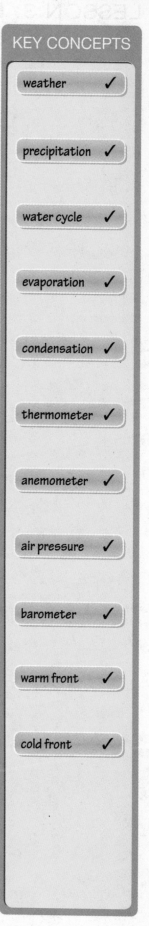

KEY CONCEPTS

weather ✓

precipitation ✓

water cycle ✓

evaporation ✓

condensation ✓

thermometer ✓

anemometer ✓

air pressure ✓

barometer ✓

warm front ✓

cold front ✓

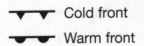

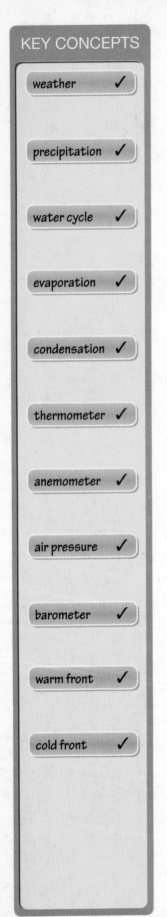

On a weather map, a warm front is marked by a line of half circles. The half circles point in the direction the front is moving. A cold front is marked by a line of triangles. The triangles point in the direction the front is heading.

Look at this weather map. Can you spot the warm fronts and the cold fronts? Which direction is each front heading?

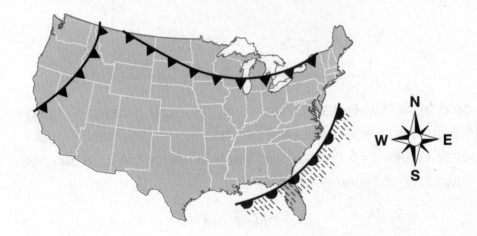

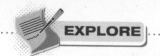 **EXPLORE**

Look at the weather map in a daily newspaper. Find your area. Is a front moving in your direction? What type is it? When is it expected? What type of weather do you think it will bring?

Pay attention to the weather for the next few days. Fill out the chart to record the change in weather that the front brings. Then compare it to what you predicted.

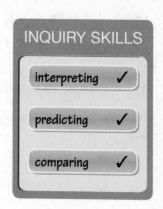

INQUIRY SKILLS

| interpreting | ✓ |
| predicting | ✓ |
| comparing | ✓ |

| TYPE OF FRONT |
| --- |
| Type of front: |
| My prediction: |
| Weather before front arrives: |
| Weather as front arrives: |
| Weather after front passes through: |

# PUTTING IT ALL TOGETHER

**You are now ready to show you understand the key concepts covered in this topic. Read each question. Circle the letter of the best answer.**

1. Where is weather made?

   A. in the ground

   B. in the air

   C. in the sea

   D. indoors

2. What is evaporation?

   A. liquid water becoming ice

   B. liquid water becoming water vapor

   C. ice becoming liquid water

   D. water vapor becoming liquid water

3. What do we call the process of water moving from Earth's surface into the air and back again?

   A. the water cycle

   B. the unicycle

   C. the weather

   D. condensation

4. What scales are used to measure temperature?

   A. only Fahrenheit

   B. only Celsius

   C. both Fahrenheit and Celsius

   D. meterstick

5. Which is an example of condensation?

   A. rain falling

   B. water freezing

   C. clouds forming

   D. water drying out

6. Which tool measures air pressure?

   A. a wind vane

   B. a water cycle

   C. a barometer

   D. an anemometer

**7.** What does an anemometer measure?

    **A.** wind speed

    **B.** air pressure

    **C.** temperature

    **D.** wind direction

**8.** What weather often occurs as a warm front approaches?

    **A.** rain becoming heavier

    **B.** rain becoming lighter

    **C.** cooler weather

    **D.** dryer weather

**Use the map to answer questions 9 and 10.**

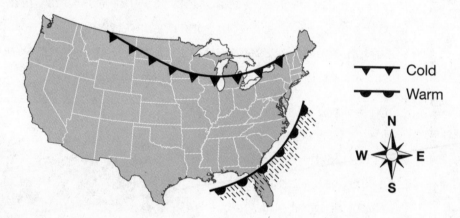

**9.** What is the line of half circles?

    **A.** a cold front

    **B.** a warm front

    **C.** low pressure

    **D.** thunderstorms

**10.** In what direction is the cold front moving?

    **A.** north

    **B.** east

    **C.** south

    **D.** west

# Forces That Change Earth's Surface

## LESSON 1: THE BASICS

**KEY CONCEPTS**

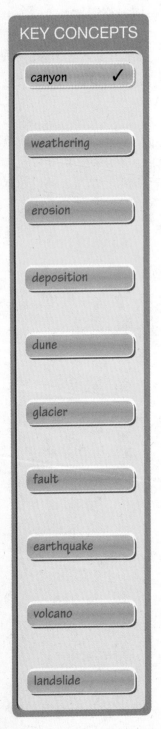

- canyon ✓
- weathering
- erosion
- deposition
- dune
- glacier
- fault
- earthquake
- volcano
- landslide

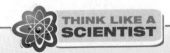

**THINK LIKE A SCIENTIST**

Summer vacation is here at last! You and your family are on a trip to the Grand Canyon. Your eyes open wide at your first look into the canyon. You have never seen or imagined so much rock! The walls of rock are striped with layers of orange and red.

You get to ride a mule along a trail to the bottom of the canyon! From time to time, you stop to talk to your guide about what you see along the way.

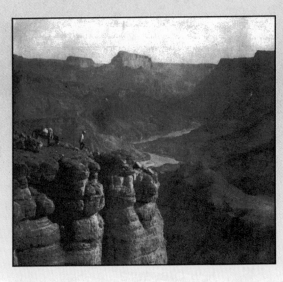

You have many questions. "This place is huge and beautiful!" you say. "How did it all get here?"

## Weathering and Erosion

Millions of years ago, this land was flat. There was no canyon here. A **canyon** is a deep, narrow valley with steep, rocky sides. But as the years passed, a canyon formed. It slowly grew deeper and steeper. Today, the Grand Canyon is 277 miles long. It is up to 15 miles wide. And it is more than a mile deep. What could have carved out this great canyon?

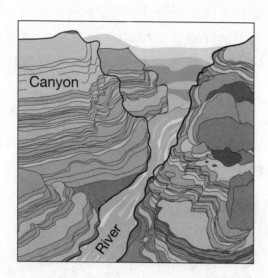

One clue you see is a blue ribbon of water at the bottom of the canyon. That ribbon is the Colorado River. Could the river have helped carve the Grand Canyon? You look around for some answers.

You notice that not everything about the Grand Canyon is big. Small pebbles, sand, and soil are all around. You guess that these small pieces of rock broke off from larger rocks.

Your guess is right. Rock being broken into smaller pieces is called **weathering**. Weathering happens when wind, water, or ice wear rock away. It also happens when plant roots get into a crack. The growing roots slowly wedge the rock apart.

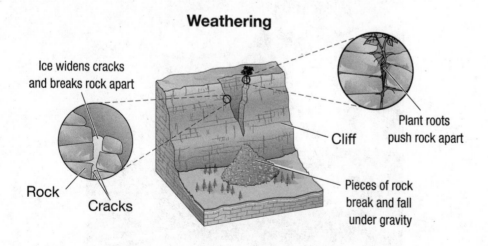

**Weathering**

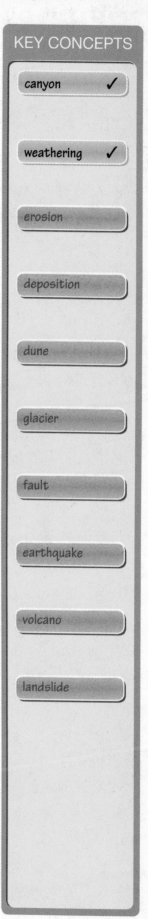

KEY CONCEPTS

- canyon ✓
- weathering ✓
- erosion
- deposition
- dune
- glacier
- fault
- earthquake
- volcano
- landslide

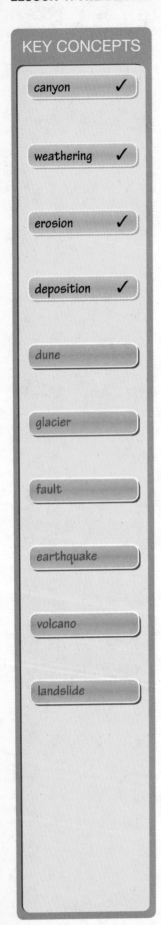

KEY CONCEPTS

canyon ✓

weathering ✓

erosion ✓

deposition ✓

dune

glacier

fault

earthquake

volcano

landslide

Over time, rock pieces fall down the canyon's side. Many of them end up in the river. The river's powerful flow moves the rocks that fall into it. The moving of rock from one place to another is called **erosion**.

What happens to all these rocks? They get dropped (or deposited) where the river slows down. That's why this process is called **deposition**.

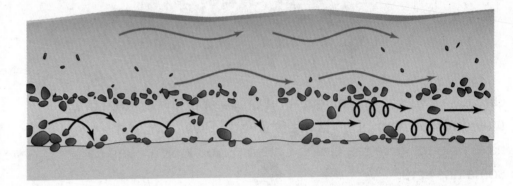

The rock pieces move with the water. They scrape against the river's bottom. This breaks pieces of rock off the bottom. These pieces are carried away by the water. The canyon grows deeper.

You look down at the rushing waters of the Colorado River. And you realize that this is the force that carved the Grand Canyon.

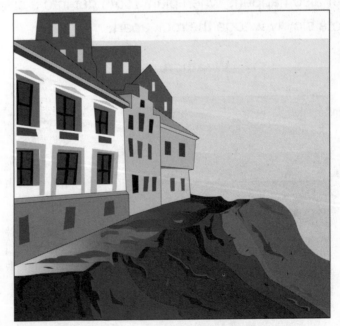

Weathering and erosion change the land all over Earth.
They can happen in your neighborhood, too.

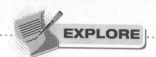

Look at the pictures below. Think about the differences between **weathering**, **erosion**, and **deposition**. Draw a line from each picture to the correct description of the earth-shaping process. Circle the name of the process.

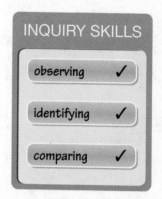

INQUIRY SKILLS

observing    ✓

identifying    ✓

comparing    ✓

| IDENTIFYING WEATHERING, EROSION, AND DEPOSITION ||
|---|---|
| 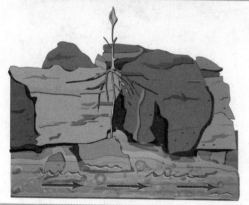 | Earth material is deposited in a new place.<br><br>weathering    erosion    deposition |
| 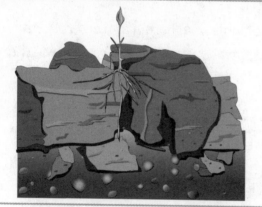 | Smaller pieces of rock break off from larger pieces.<br><br>weathering    erosion    deposition |
| 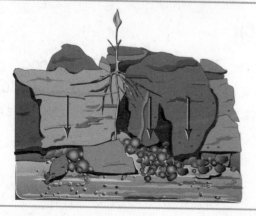 | Earth material is moved from one place to another.<br><br>weathering    erosion    deposition |

# LESSON 2: **BUILDING ON THE BASICS**

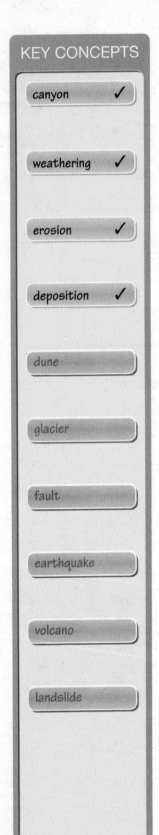

## KEY CONCEPTS

canyon ✓

weathering ✓

erosion ✓

deposition ✓

dune

glacier

fault

earthquake

volcano

landslide

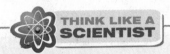
**THINK LIKE A SCIENTIST**

What an exciting day! But you are tired. It took you six hours to ride your mule to the bottom of the canyon. Now you get to camp overnight near the Colorado River.

Settled in your sleeping bag, you listen to the river. You hear the rustle of leaves in the nearby brush. You feel the breeze on your cheek. In the moonlight, you see that the wind is blowing tiny grains of sand along the ground right beside your pillow.

Your guide says that even tonight, weathering and erosion are making the Grand Canyon deeper. You wonder, "How much will the canyon change around me while I sleep?"

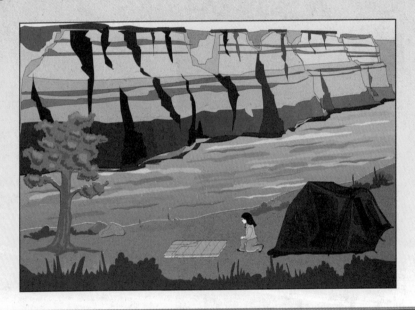

## Slow Changes to Earth

The Grand Canyon changes very little in one day. Weathering, erosion, and deposition take a long time to change the land. Most changes to Earth's surface are slow. They happen so slowly that we do not even notice them.

## Water

Moving water can slowly cut a canyon through rock. You have seen the results of that with your own eyes. What else can cause such slow changes?

## Wind

Wind can slowly wear away rock. It can also slowly build new land. One way it builds new land is by piling up small pieces of rock, like sand. In dry, flat places, the wind can build sand dunes. A **dune** is a pile of sand. You will find dunes in deserts and at the back of beaches.

You've probably never seen a dune move. But it can! Sand blows up one side of the dune. Then the sand falls down the other side. As the wind keeps blowing, the dune is worn away on one side. It is built up on the other side. The drawing shows how a dune can move from right to left.

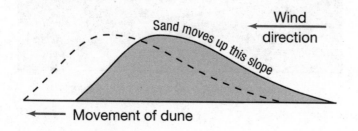

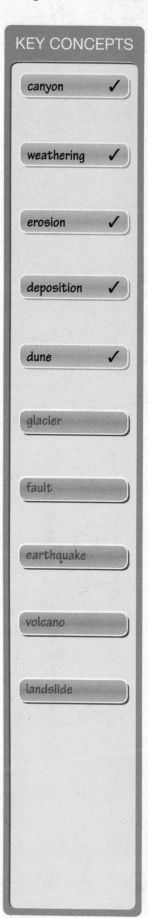

KEY CONCEPTS

canyon ✓

weathering ✓

erosion ✓

deposition ✓

dune ✓

glacier

fault

earthquake

volcano

landslide

147

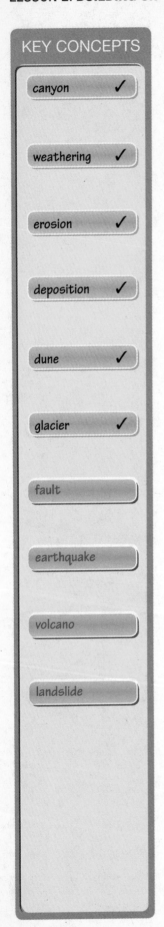

# Ice

Moving ice can also slowly change Earth's surface. A glacier is a large sheet of moving ice. A **glacier** forms from snow that has piled up on a mountain. The weight of the snow turns it into ice. As you might guess, a glacier moves downhill. It is like a slowly moving river of ice. The moving glacier scrapes away rocks and soil under it.

Many years later, a warmer climate may melt the glacier. It will disappear. But it will leave behind the valleys it has carved. And it may leave behind huge holes in the ground. The holes may fill with water to make lakes. The Great Lakes in the northern United States were made this way.

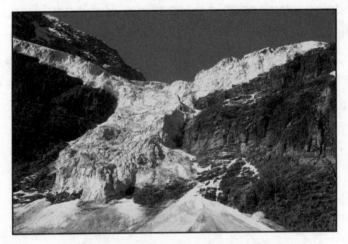

A glacier changes the land it moves over.

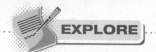 **EXPLORE**

Create a complete sentence from each word group below. Next, tell how each sentence is an example of weathering, erosion, and/or deposition.

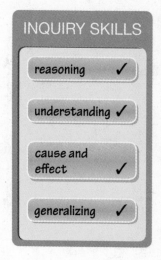

INQUIRY SKILLS

reasoning ✓

understanding ✓

cause and effect ✓

generalizing ✓

| Word Group | Your Sentence | How Is This Weathering, Erosion, and/or Deposition? |
|---|---|---|
| water canyon rocks and pebbles | | |
| wind dune sand | | |
| ice glacier rocks | | |

## KEY CONCEPTS

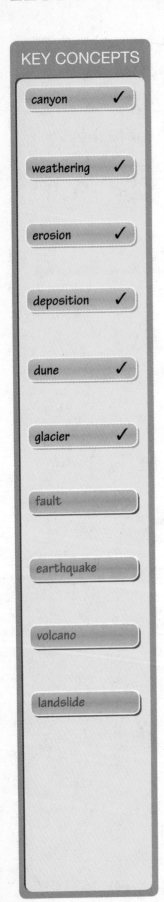

- canyon ✓
- weathering ✓
- erosion ✓
- deposition ✓
- dune ✓
- glacier ✓
- fault
- earthquake
- volcano
- landslide

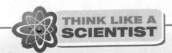

**THINK LIKE A SCIENTIST**

Your airplane lifts into the sky. Your vacation is over and it's time to head to your home in California.

In the Grand Canyon, you discovered how land can be changed slowly. But you wonder, "Can land also be changed quickly? And, if it can, by what?"

About an hour into your flight, you look down. You see a curious sight. The land seems to be split by a long crack. All of a sudden, you remember what that crack is. And you realize it's a clue to the answer to your questions.

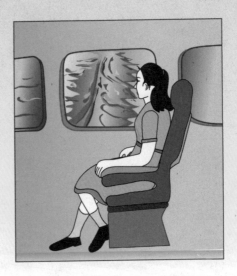

## Fast Changes to Earth

You recognize the "crack." It's the San Andreas Fault. But what is a fault? And what does it have to do with quick changes in the land?

A **fault** is a long, deep crack in Earth's crust. Land sometimes moves suddenly along a fault. The land may move up, down, sideways, or apart. When it moves, it sets off an earthquake. An **earthquake** is the shaking of the ground. An earthquake can quickly change the shape of the land.

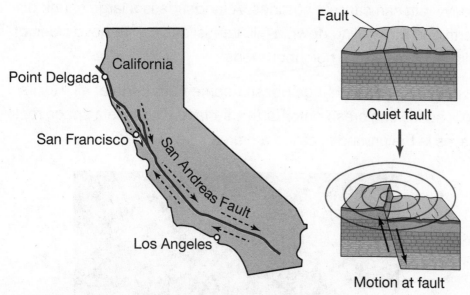

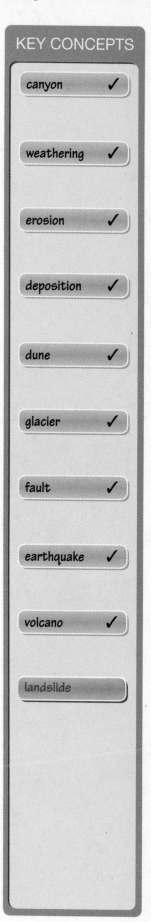

KEY CONCEPTS

canyon ✓

weathering ✓

erosion ✓

deposition ✓

dune ✓

glacier ✓

fault ✓

earthquake ✓

volcano ✓

landslide

The San Andreas Fault is in California. Many earthquakes have happened along this fault.

Most volcanoes form near faults. A **volcano** is an opening where melted rock comes up from deep beneath the ground. The melted rock can flow smoothly from a hole in Earth's surface. Then it cools and hardens. This builds new land. It builds a mountain. But sometimes after the mountain forms, the melted rock can blow it up. So the melted rock destroys a mountain, or part of one.

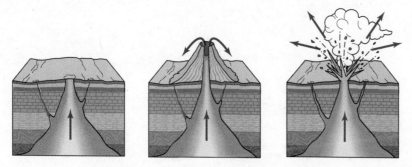

A volcano can build up or break down land.

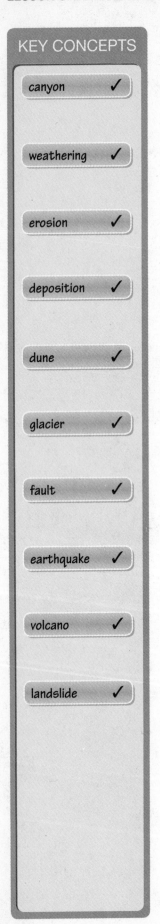

KEY CONCEPTS

- canyon ✓
- weathering ✓
- erosion ✓
- deposition ✓
- dune ✓
- glacier ✓
- fault ✓
- earthquake ✓
- volcano ✓
- landslide ✓

Volcanoes and earthquakes cause fast changes to Earth's surface. These changes come from forces inside the planet. Other fast changes come from forces above Earth's surface. For example, big storms can cause fast changes. A really big storm, like a hurricane, can wash away a whole beach in just a few hours.

Heavy rain can cause landslides. A **landslide** is a large chunk of earth and rock falling down a hill. Landslides can remove sides of hills as big as whole neighborhoods.

Sometimes, a fast change doesn't come from Earth at all. Rocks from space can crash onto Earth's surface. The hole a space rock leaves in the ground is called a *crater*.

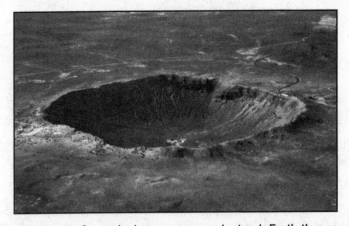

This crater was formed when a space rock struck Earth thousands of years ago. It is located in Arizona. The crater is as deep as a 57-story building is tall. It's as wide as 11 soccer fields are long.

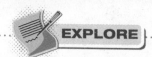 **EXPLORE**

Find two books of the same thickness that you can lay flat next to each other. Also find three or four smaller flat-sided objects that you can stack on top of the books. (You can use blocks, erasers, or anything that is smaller than the books and flat enough to stack.)

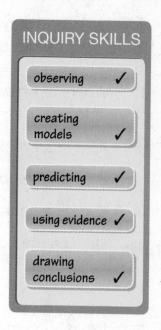

INQUIRY SKILLS

| observing | ✓ |
| creating models | ✓ |
| predicting | ✓ |
| using evidence | ✓ |
| drawing conclusions | ✓ |

| CREATE A MODEL OF MOVING LAND | |
|---|---|
| Place two books flat on your desk next to each other. Line the books up so their edges are flat against each other. | |
| If your two books were pieces of land, what would you call the line between them where they touch each other? | |
| Next, build a stack of the three or four smaller objects across the line between your books. | |
| What does your stack of smaller objects represent in your model? | |
| What do you expect to happen if you move one of the books? | |
| Now, slide one of your books forward on your desk while you hold the other book still. | |
| What have you just created a model of? | |
| What happened to your building? What can happen to real buildings when the land beneath them moves? | |

# PUTTING IT ALL TOGETHER

You are now ready to show you understand the key concepts covered in this topic. Read each question. Circle the letter of the best answer.

1. Where is a glacier MOST LIKELY to form?

   A. in a hot desert

   B. on a mountain

   C. in a thick forest

   D. on the floor of a canyon

2. What happens when huge pieces of land suddenly slide up, down, sideways, or apart?

   A. erosion

   B. a flood

   C. weathering

   D. an earthquake

3. Which means the breaking down of rock into smaller pieces?

   A. weathering

   B. erosion

   C. eruption

   D. sliding

4. What happens along faults?

   A. earthquakes

   B. glaciers

   C. erosion

   D. canyons

5. When is a sand dune MOST LIKELY to move?

   A. when it is hot

   B. when it is cold

   C. when the wind is slow

   D. when the wind is fast

6. Which force changes Earth's surface slowly?

   A. landslide

   B. earthquake

   C. volcano

   D. glacier

7. What dug the Grand Canyon?

    A. air

    B. melted rock

    C. ice

    D. water

8. How will the Grand Canyon probably change in the future?

    A. It will fill in.

    B. It will get deeper.

    C. It will move sideways.

    D. It will get wider.

9. Which word BEST describes how the Grand Canyon formed?

    A. erosion

    B. explosion

    C. fault

    D. volcano

10. Which BEST describes a glacier?

    A. a river of ice

    B. a layer of ice

    C. a lake of ice

    D. a mountain of ice

# GLOSSARY

**adaptation** a trait that helps a living thing to survive (page 86)

**air pressure** the weight of air pressing on Earth's surface (page 134)

**anemometer** a tool that measures how fast the wind is blowing (page 133)

**axis** an imaginary line that Earth spins around. The axis goes through Earth from the North Pole to the South Pole. (page 115)

**balance** a tool used for measuring mass (page 68)

**barometer** a tool that measures air pressure (page 134)

**canyon** a deep, narrow valley with steep sides (page 142)

**characteristic** something that identifies an object or a living thing. It can be part of the object, or something it does. (page 101)

**chemical energy** energy stored inside material (page 77)

**climate** average weather in an area over a long time period (page 90)

**cold front** a fast-moving weather front that is followed by cooler air (page 137)

**conclusion** the last step in an experiment; a decision you make based on how you interpreted your data (page 40)

**condensation** water vapor in the air changing into liquid water or ice (page 130)

**consumer** a living thing that gets energy by eating plants or animals (page 109)

**control** to keep a variable from changing during an experiment (page 22)

**crescent** a curved shape that is thick in the middle and pointed on its ends (page 124)

**data** a group of facts and observations recorded during an experiment (pages 26, 32)

**day** one rotation of Earth (page 116)

**decomposer** a living thing that gets energy from dead plants or animals (page 109)

**deposition** the dropping of material, such as pieces of rock, in new places (page 144)

**direction** the path taken as something moves (page 50)

**distance** how far something moves (page 48)

**dune** a large pile of sand built up by the wind (page 147)

**earthquake** shaking of the ground (page 151)

**electrical energy** energy in the form of electricity. Electrical energy comes from the tiny, moving particles that make up matter. (page 78)

**energy** the ability to do work or cause change  (page 73)

**environment** all of the living and nonliving things that surround a living thing  (page 100)

**erosion** the moving of material such as rock by natural forces  (page 144)

**evaporation** liquid water changing into water vapor and entering the air  (page 130)

**experiment** a controlled test  (pages 21, 30)

**extinct** gone forever  (page 92)

**fault** a long crack in Earth's crust. Parts of Earth slide past each other at faults.  (page 151)

**food chain** the way food moves from one living thing to another  (page 110)

**food web** a group of connected food chains, showing different ways food moves through an environment  (page 110)

**force** any push or pull  (page 45)

**fossil** any evidence of ancient life  (page 95)

**gas** a form of matter in which particles are not connected and can move about freely  (page 64)

**glacier** a large sheet of ice that forms from snow. Gravity makes glaciers flow down mountains.  (page 148)

**graph** a way to show data. A graph shows how one thing changes as another thing changes.  (page 35)

**heat energy** energy that makes something warm  (page 76)

**hemisphere** half of Earth. Earth has a Northern Hemisphere and a Southern Hemisphere.  (page 119)

**hypothesis** a guess that you can test  (page 20)

**interpret data** to look carefully at a collection of facts to figure out what they mean  (page 38)

**kinetic energy** energy that is doing work or causing change  (page 74)

**landslide** a large mass of earth and rock crashing down a slope  (page 152)

**length** the distance from one end of a solid to the other  (page 67)

**liquid** a form of matter in which particles are loosely connected and can move past each other  (page 64)

**machine** something that makes work easier  (page 53)

**mass** the amount of matter in an object  (page 59)

**matter** anything that has weight and takes up space  (page 59)

**mechanical energy** the energy of motion  (page 77)

**moon phases** the different shapes that the moon appears to take as it revolves (page 123)

**motion** a change in the position of an object (page 45)

**observation** using your senses to notice facts about something (page 17)

**pattern** a regular change in the data (page 39)

**photosynthesis** the way plants use sunlight, air, and water to make food (page 106)

**physical properties** traits of an object that can be observed (page 59)

**precipitation** falling rain, sleet, hail, or snow (page 129)

**predator** an animal that eats other animals (page 109)

**prey** the animal that a predator hunts and eats (page 109)

**producer** a living thing that makes its own food (page 109)

**potential energy** energy that is ready to be used (page 74)

**record** to keep track of observations (page 18)

**reproduce** make more of one's own kind (page 101)

**revolution** the movement of Earth around the sun. It takes Earth one year to make one revolution. (page 118)

**rotation** Earth's spinning motion (page 115)

**season** a part of the year with a certain kind of weather. Fall, winter, spring, and summer are seasons. (page 118)

**senses** sight, hearing, smell, taste, and touch. You use your senses to observe physical properties of matter. (page 60)

**simple machine** a tool that makes it easier to move an object (page 53)

**solid** a form of matter in which particles are packed close together. A solid has a definite shape. (page 63)

**speed** how fast something moves (page 49)

**survive** stay alive (page 109)

**table** a chart for listing numbers and facts. A table has columns and rows. (page 34)

**thermal energy** energy that makes you feel warm. Thermal energy is sometimes called heat. (page 80)

**thermometer** a tool that measures temperature (page 132)

**variable** something that can change during an experiment. A good experiment only allows one variable to change at a time. (page 22)

**volcano** an opening where lava erupts from beneath the ground (page 151)

**volume** the amount of space that an object takes up (page 67)

**warm front** a weather front that often pushes clouds and rain ahead of it. Warmer weather follows when the front has passed. (page 137)

**water cycle** movement of water from the land and sea into the air, and back again (page 130)

**weather** the state of the air at a given place and time (page 128)

**weathering** the process of wind, water, or ice wearing rock away (page 143)

**work** the use of force to move an object (page 52)

**year** the time it takes for Earth to make one revolution around the sun (page 118)